Medical Management of Non-Insulin-Dependent (Type II) Diabetes

Third Edition

D0932974

American Diabetes Association

CLINICAL EDUCATION SERIES

Chief Scientific and Medical Officer
Richard Kahn, PhD

Publisher
Susan H. Lau

Editorial Director
Peter Banks

Managing Editor
Christine B. Welch

Associate Editor
Sherrye Landrum

Director of Production
Carolyn R. Segree

American Diabetes Association, Inc., Alexandria, VA 22314
© 1994 by the American Diabetes Association, Inc. All rights reserved.
First printing June 1994
Printed in the United States of America
ISBN 0-945448-37-6

Contents

iii

A Word About This Guide

The *Medical Management of Non-Insulin-Dependent (Type II) Diabetes* is the most recent addition to the American Diabetes Association's Clinical Education Series, which also includes *Medical Management of Insulin-Dependent (Type I) Diabetes, Therapy for Diabetes Mellitus and Related Disorders*, and *Medical Management of Pregnancy Complicated by Diabetes*. The Clinical Education Series was designed to provide health care professionals with the comprehensive information needed to give the best possible medical care to patients with diabetes mellitus.

This book evolved from the *Physician's Guide to Non-Insulin-Dependent (Type II) Diabetes: Diagnosis and Treatment*. New information has improved our knowledge about the pathogenesis of diabetes. Although the landmark Diabetes Control and Complications Trial demonstrated the value of glycemic control in patients with type I diabetes, many experts believe its findings have implications for the treatment of type II diabetes as well. Finally, in 1994, the American Diabetes Association issued revised position statements on *Standards of Medical Care for Patients With Diabetes Mellitus* and *Nutrition Recommendations and Principles for People With Diabetes Mellitus*. These hallmark clinical practice recommendations have been incorporated into this text.

It is clear that proper nutrition, exercise, and excellent blood glucose regulation in addition to attention to blood pressure and lipid levels are key elements in the management of type II diabetes. The development of *Medical Management of Non-Insulin-Dependent (Type II) Diabetes* was designed to provide state-of-the-art information on these issues. Its publication could not have been possible without the expert guidance of the many contributors to the first, second, and present editions. The book's focus on pathogenesis, diagnosis and classification, routine management, and maintaining wellness through proper nutrition, exercise, and the treatment of complications was the work of many experts, who laid this comprehensive foundation in the book's previous editions. In particular, we are indebted to the editors-in-chief of the first and second editions, Harold Rifkin, MD, and Harold E. Lebovitz, MD.

The American Diabetes Association believes that you will find this book as useful as its predecessors. Hopefully, it will encourage you to add other American Diabetes Association publications to your library, which can help you manage your patients with diabetes more effectively.

PHILIP RASKIN, MD
Editor-in-Chief

Contributors

Editor-in-Chief

PHILIP RASKIN, MD
University of Texas Southwestern Medical Center
Dallas, Texas

Contributing
Editors

CHRISTINE A. BEEBE, MS, BS, RD
St. James Hospital and Health Center
Chicago Heights, Illinois

MAYER B. DAVIDSON, MD
Cedars-Sinai Medical Center
Los Angeles, California

DAVID NATHAN, MD
Massachusetts General Hospital
Boston, Massachusetts

ROBERT A. RIZZA, MD
Mayo Clinic
Rochester, Minnesota

ROBERT SHERWIN, MD
Yale School of Medicine
New Haven, Connecticut

Reviewers

GERALD BERNSTEIN, MD
Montefiore Medical Center
Bronx, New York

CHARLES M. CLARK, JR., MD
Indiana University School of Medicine
Indianapolis, Indiana

JOHN A. COLWELL, MD, PhD
Medical University of South Carolina
Charleston, South Carolina

ANNE DALY, MS, RD, CDE
Springfield Diabetes and Endocrine Center
Springfield, Illinois

JOHN T. DEVLIN, MD
Maine Medical Center
Portland, Maine

BORIS DRAZNIN, MD, PhD
Department of Veterans Affairs Medical Center
Denver, Colorado

ALLEN J. GARBER, MD, PhD
Baylor Collge of Medicine
Houston, Texas

LAWRENCE B. HARKLESS, DPM
University of Texas Health Sciences Center
San Antonio, Texas

C. RONALD KAHN, MD
Joslin Diabetes Center
Boston, Massachusetts

CAROLYN LEONTOS, MS, RD, CDE
University of Nevada
Las Vegas, Nevada

DEREK LeROITH, MD, PhD
National Institutes of Health
Bethesda, Maryland

ERNEST L. MAZZAFERRI, MD
The Ohio State University Hospitals
Columbus, Ohio

MARK E. MOLITCH, MD
Northwestern University School of Medicine
Chicago, Illinois

RONALD P. MONSAERT, MD
Geisinger Medical Center
Danville, Pennsylvania

STEPHEN H. SCHNEIDER, MD
Robert Wood Johnson Medical School
New Brunswick, New Jersey

HARRY SHAMOON, MD
Albert Einstein College of Medicine
Bronx, New York

JAY S. SKYLER, MD
University of Miami
Miami, Florida

PATRICIA D. STENGER, RN, CDE
Eastern Maine Medical Center
Bangor, Maine

KARL E. SUSSMAN, MD
Department of Veterans Affairs Medical Center
Denver, Colorado

ELIZABETH A. WALKER, RN, DNSc, CDE
Albert Einstein College of Medicine
Bronx, New York

Diagnosis and Classification

Highlights
Diagnosis and Classification

Diabetes mellitus is a disorder characterized by fasting hyperglycemia or plasma glucose levels above defined limits during oral glucose tolerance testing. The classification of diabetes mellitus and other categories of glucose intolerance includes three clinical classes: diabetes mellitus, impaired glucose tolerance (IGT), and gestational diabetes mellitus (GDM), and four clinical subclasses of diabetes mellitus:

■ insulin-dependent diabetes mellitus (type I or IDDM):~10% of known cases of diabetes in the United States are type I.

■ non-insulin-dependent diabetes mellitus (type II or NIDDM): ~90% of all known cases of diabetes in the United States are type II.

■ secondary diabetes mellitus: patients with other types of diabetes mellitus have unusual causes of diabetes due to certain diseases of the pancreas, hormonal syndromes, drugs, rare conditions involving the insulin receptor, and other genetic syndromes.

■ malnutrition-related diabetes mellitus: occurs mostly in developing countries in young, obviously lean individuals.

Patients with IGT have plasma glucose levels that are higher than normal but not diagnostic for diabetes mellitus. About 25% of patients with IGT eventually develop diabetes mellitus.

Patients with GDM have onset or discovery of glucose intolerance during pregnancy, usually in the 2nd or 3rd trimester.

Distinguishing characteristics of these categories of glucose intolerance are summarized in Table 1.1.

Candidates for screening tests include
■ people with 1st-degree relatives with diabetes mellitus,
■ people who are markedly obese,
■ individuals of certain races (American Indian, Hispanic, or African American),
■ individuals >40 yr of age and any of the preceding factors,
■ women with previous GDM or a history of babies >9 lb at birth,
■ all pregnant women between 24 and 28 wk of pregnancy,
■ individuals with hypertension or hyperlipidemias, and
■ individuals with previously identified IGT.

Criteria for positive screening tests are summarized in Table 1.4.

Indications for diagnostic testing include
■ positive screening test results,
■ obvious signs and symptoms of diabetes mellitus (polydipsia, polyuria, polyphagia, weight loss), and
■ an incomplete clinical picture, such as glucosuria or equivocal elevation of random plasma glucose level.

Criteria for diagnosis of diabetes mellitus, impaired glucose tolerance, and gestational diabetes are summarized in Table 1.5.

Before treatment, a complete evaluation should be made to determine
■ the type of diabetes or glucose intolerance,
■ the presence of underlying diseases that need further evaluation, and
■ the presence of complications.

Diagnosis and Classification

INTRODUCTION

Diabetes mellitus is a chronic disorder characterized by abnormalities in the metabolism of carbohydrate, protein, and fat; it is often accompanied, after some time, by microvascular, macrovascular, and neuropathic complications. It is now recognized that diabetes mellitus encompasses a group of genetically and clinically heterogeneous disorders in which glucose intolerance is a common denominator. Thus, although diabetes mellitus affects the metabolism of all body fuels, its diagnosis depends on identification of specific plasma glucose abnormalities.

Because the syndrome of diabetes mellitus encompasses many disorders that differ in pathogenesis, natural history, and responses to treatment, it is important that clinicians and researchers use commonly accepted terminology as well as standardized classification and diagnostic criteria when categorizing patients with glucose intolerance.

TYPES OF DIABETES MELLITUS AND OTHER CATEGORIES OF GLUCOSE INTOLERANCE

The classification of diabetes mellitus and other categories of glucose intolerance (Table 1.1) includes three clinical classes: diabetes mellitus, impaired glucose tolerance (IGT), and gestational diabetes mellitus (GDM), and four clinical subclasses of diabetes mellitus.

Diabetes Mellitus

The term *diabetes mellitus* is applied to disorders characterized by fasting hyperglycemia or plasma glucose levels above defined limits. There are four clinical subclasses of diabetes mellitus, each of which has distinguishing characteristics:
- insulin-dependent (type I) diabetes mellitus
- non-insulin-dependent (type II) diabetes mellitus
- secondary and other types of diabetes (diabetes mellitus associated with certain conditions and syndromes), and
- malnutrition-related diabetes mellitus.

Type I diabetes. Patients with type I diabetes mellitus have severe insulinopenia and are prone to the development of ketoacidosis. Commonly, type I patients are lean and have experienced recent weight loss. By definition, patients with this type of diabetes mellitus are dependent on exogenous insulin to prevent ketoacidosis and death. Type I diabetes is less frequent among some nonwhite populations and is estimated to account for ~10% of all known cases of diabetes mellitus in the United States. Although type I diabetes may occur at any age, the major peak of onset occurs at about 11 or 12 yr, and nearly all patients diagnosed before age 20 are of this type. However, while exact prevalence remains to be established, many Hispanic and African American youths with onset of diabetes before age 20 have type II diabetes.

The etiology of type I diabetes mellitus involves immunologic destruction of the β-cells. It appears, however, that it is a heterogeneous disorder in terms of precipitating events. Genetic factors are important because there is a clear association between type I diabetes and certain histocompatibility locus antigens (HLA) on chromosome 6. Also, identical twin studies indicate that only 25–50% of identical twins of type I patients develop the disease, suggesting both a genetic and environmental etiology for the disease. That type I diabetes is an autoimmune disease is suggested by the observation that the majority of patients have circulating antibodies to islet cells, to endogenous insulin, and/or to other antigens that are constituents of islet cells at the time of diagnosis. The nature of environmental factors that may contribute to the etiology of the disease remains unknown. One attractive hypothesis is that a viral infection stimulates an autoimmune reaction through molecular mimicry in genetically susceptible individuals.

Table 1.1. Types of Diabetes Mellitus and Other Categories of Abnormal Glucose Metabolism

CLINICAL CLASSES	DISTINGUISHING CHARACTERISTICS
Diabetes mellitus Insulin-dependent diabetes mellitus (IDDM or type I)	Patients may be of any age, are not usually obese, and often have abrupt onset of signs and symptoms with insulinopenia before age 30. These patients often have strongly positive urine ketone tests in conjunction with hyperglycemia and are dependent on insulin therapy to prevent ketoacidosis and to sustain life.
Non-insulin-dependent diabetes mellitus (NIDDM or type II) (obese or nonobese)	Patients usually are >30 yr at diagnosis, obese, and have relatively few classic symptoms. They are not prone to ketoacidosis except during periods of stress. Although not dependent on exogenous insulin for survival, they may require it for adequate control of hyperglycemia.
Secondary and other types of diabetes	Patients with secondary and other types of diabetes mellitus have certain associated conditions or syndromes (see Table 1.2).
Malnutrition-related diabetes mellitus*	Patients are young (between 10 and 40 yr old), usually symptomatic, and not prone to ketoacidosis, but most require insulin therapy.
Impaired glucose tolerance (IGT) (obese or nonobese)	Patients with impaired glucose tolerance have plasma glucose levels that are higher than normal but not diagnostic for diabetes mellitus.
Gestational diabetes mellitus (GDM)	Patients with gestational diabetes mellitus have onset or discovery of glucose intolerance during pregnancy.

*Recommended as a separate clinical class of diabetes mellitus by the World Health Organization (WHO); see Bibliography.
Adapted from classification developed by an international work group sponsored by the National Diabetes Data Group, National Institutes of Health; see Bibliography.

Type II diabetes. Patients with type II diabetes mellitus have residual insulin secretory capacity although insulin levels are inadequate to overcome the concomitant insulin resistance, and hyperglycemia ensues. Commonly, these patients are obese and may not experience classic symptoms of uncontrolled diabetes. Type II diabetes is more common in individuals of nonwhite descent. It is characterized as follows:

■ Type II diabetes can occur at any age but is usually diagnosed after age 30.
■ Although about 80% of patients are obese or have a history of obesity at the time of diagnosis, type II diabetes can occur in nonobese individuals as well, especially in the elderly.
■ Patients with type II diabetes may or may not present with classic symptoms of diabetes mellitus (polydipsia, polyuria, polyphagia, weight loss).
■ Patients with type II diabetes are not prone to develop ketoacidosis except during periods or conditions of severe stress, such as those caused by infections, trauma, or surgery.
■ Patients with type II diabetes may present with microvascular and

macrovascular chronic complications.

■ Type II diabetes is associated with defects in both insulin secretion and insulin action.

Although patients with type II diabetes are not dependent on exogenous insulin for survival, many patients require insulin for adequate glycemic control. Insulin may also be needed temporarily for control of stress-induced hyperglycemia.

Type II diabetes accounts for about 90% of the diabetic patients in the United States. The prevalence of diagnosed type II diabetes mellitus in the United States is about 7 million people, or roughly 3% of the population. There is, most likely, an equal number of undiagnosed cases. The prevalence of type II diabetes is markedly increased among American Indians, African Americans, and Hispanics. The prevalence rate increases with age and degree of obesity. There is evidence that the number of new cases diagnosed each year is increasing.

The etiology of type II diabetes mellitus remains unknown. It appears to be a heterogeneous disorder, and both genetic and environmental factors are important. Although type II diabetes mellitus is not associated with specific HLA tissue types, identical twin studies indicate that there is 58–75% concordance for this disease. There are families in which type II diabetes is present in children, adolescents, and adults and in which an autosomal dominant inheritance has been established. This form of diabetes is referred to as *maturity-onset diabetes of the young* (MODY). In many (but not all) of these families, various abnormalities have been found in the gene coding for glucokinase, an enzyme important for glucose-induced insulin secretion and glucose uptake by the liver. Unlike type I diabetes, circulating islet cell antibodies are rarely present. Intake of excessive calories leading to weight gain and obesity is probably an important factor in the pathogenesis of type II diabetes. In fact, obesity has been singled out as a most powerful risk factor, and even small weight losses are associated with a change in plasma glucose levels toward normal in many patients with this type of diabetes.

Secondary and other types of diabetes. This category, which is numerically the smallest, includes diabetes mellitus associated with certain diseases, drugs, or conditions. To be placed in this category, the patient's diabetes either has a known or probable cause or is part of a specific condition or syndrome. Table 1.2 presents the several subclasses of this category.

Malnutrition-related diabetes. Another category of diabetes that is seen in developing countries is malnutrition-related diabetes mellitus. Afflicted individuals are usually young (between 10 and 40 yr old). They are symptomatic with marked polyuria, polydipsia, and weight loss. Insulin is usually required to control their hyperglycemia, although they remain ketosis-resistant even when insulin is withdrawn. Some of these patients experience antecedent abdominal pain radiating to the back, suggesting pancreatitis. Indeed, some show pancreatic calcifications on radiography, and at autopsy, endocrine destruction and fibrosis as well as calcium stones in the exocrine ducts are seen. However, chronic pancreatitis does not account for malnutrition-related diabetes because insulin requirements are high (patients with diabetes secondary to pancreatic inflammation are usually sensitive to insulin), and many of these patients have no clinical or autopsy evidence of pancreatitis. The role of malnutrition in causing this kind of diabetes is unknown. This type of diabetes mellitus seems mostly confined to developing countries.

Impaired Glucose Tolerance

IGT is the term used to describe individuals who have plasma glucose levels that are higher than normal but lower than those considered diagnostic for diabetes mellitus. Patients in this category may be subgrouped by weight (obese and nonobese) (Table 1.1). Those with IGT secondary to or associated with certain conditions and syndromes consti-

Table 1.2. Secondary Diabetes Mellitus and Impaired Glucose Tolerance

SECONDARY TO:

Pancreatic disease	Examples: pancreatectomy, hemochromatosis, cystic fibrosis, chronic pancreatitis
Endocrinopathies	Examples: Cushing's syndrome, acromegaly pheochromocytoma, primary aldosteronism, glucagonoma
Drugs and chemical agents	Examples: certain antihypertensive drugs, thiazide diuretics, glucocorticoids, estrogen-containing preparations, nicotinic acid, phenytoin, catecholamines

ASSOCIATED WITH:

Insulin receptor abnormalities	Example: acanthosis nigricans
Genetic syndromes	Examples: lipodrystophic syndromes, muscular dystrophies, Huntington's chorea
Miscellaneous conditions	Example: polycystic ovary disease

For a more complete list, see National Diabetes Data Group, in Bibliography.

tute another subgroup (Table 1.2). Approximately 25% of patients with IGT eventually develop diabetes mellitus. Although patients with IGT do not appear to have an increased risk for the microvascular complications of diabetes mellitus, they have been shown in some populations to have a greater than normal risk for atherosclerotic disease.

Gestational Diabetes Mellitus

The term GDM is used to describe glucose intolerance that has its onset or is first detected during pregnancy. Women with known diabetes mellitus before conception are not part of this class. GDM occurs in about 2–4% of pregnant women, usually during the second or third trimester, when levels of insulin-antagonist hormones increase and insulin resistance normally occurs. Because fetal morbidity is increased in the presence of GDM, it is important to identify women with this condition by performing screening tests in all pregnant women between the 24th and 28th wk of pregnancy.

After parturition, patients with GDM should be followed closely. In most cases, glucose tolerance in women with GDM returns to normal after delivery. Within 5–15 yr after parturition, however, 40–60% of women with GDM develop type II diabetes mellitus.

DIAGNOSIS OF DIABETES MELLITUS AND OTHER CATEGORIES OF GLUCOSE INTOLERANCE

The prevalence of undiagnosed diabetes mellitus in the United States is about 3% of the population, and the currently recommended diagnostic tests for diabetes are neither 100% specific nor 100% sensitive. Based on these facts, it is generally agreed that the risk to the patient of inappropriate diagnosis outweighs the benefits to be gained from screening tests for diabetes in the general community. However, screening high-risk individuals (see list below) may be appropriate.

Indications and Criteria for Evaluation for Diabetes Mellitus

The recommended screening test for nonpregnant adults is a fasting plasma glucose determination. Evaluation for diabetes mellitus should be limited to nonpregnant individuals with a high risk of developing diabetes. High-risk candidates include:

■ people with 1st-degree relatives with diabetes mellitus,
■ people who are obese (>20% over desirable body weight),
■ individuals of certain races (American Indian, Hispanic, or African American),
■ individuals >40 yr of age plus any of the preceding factors,
■ individuals with hypertension or hyperlipidemia,
■ individuals with previously identified IGT,
■ all pregnant women at 24–28 wk of pregnancy, and
■ women with previous GDM or a history of delivering a baby weighing >9 lb.

It is particularly important to screen all pregnant women for the presence of GDM because 60,000–90,000 women with the disease give birth each year, and GDM is associated with increased perinatal morbidity. In pregnant women, a 50-g oral glucose load is recommended for screening. Normal plasma glucose values are presented in Table 1.3, and criteria for positive screening tests are presented in Table 1.4. Individuals with plasma glucose levels <115 mg/dl (<6.4 mM) should be rescreened in 3 yr if they still have one or more of the risk factors listed above.

Diagnostic Tests for Diabetes Mellitus

Diagnostic tests for diabetes should be done if a patient has a positive screening test or obvious signs and symptoms of diabetes, e.g., polydipsia, polyuria, polyphagia, or weight loss. A diagnosis can be made on the basis of a random plasma glucose concentration plus signs and symptoms of diabetes, a fasting plasma glucose concentration, or a properly performed oral glucose tolerance test (OGTT). Although urine glucose tests are strongly suggestive of diabetes in symptomatic patients, they should never be used for the diagnosis of diabetes mellitus. The choice of diagnostic tests and their interpretation are different for nonpregnant adults and pregnant women (Table 1.5). In nonpregnant adults, the diagnosis of diabetes mellitus is restricted to those who have *one* of the following:

■ a random plasma glucose level ≥200 mg/dl (≥11.1 mM) plus classic signs *and* symptoms of diabetes mellitus including polydipsia, polyuria, polyphagia, and weight loss, or
■ a fasting plasma concentration ≥140 mg/dl (≥7.8 mM) on at least two occasions, or
■ a fasting plasma glucose concentration <140 mg/dl (≥7.8mM) and a 2-h glucose concentration in the OGTT ≥200 mg/dl (≥11.1 mM) (see below) on two occasions.

Certain factors elevate plasma glucose levels including certain drugs (Table 1.2), stress, marked restriction of carbohydrate intake, or prolonged physical inactivity. These must be taken into account when interpreting the results of diagnostic tests for diabetes.

Oral glucose tolerance test. The standard OGTT is often unnecessary for diagnosis of diabetes mellitus. If performed, the OGTT is useful only if done with strict adherence to proper methods (insurance of proper adequate carbohydrate diet, i.e., 150 g/day for 3 days, absence of

---

Table 1.3. Normal Plasma Glucose Values for Nonpregnant Adults

Fasting		<115 mg/dl (<6.4 mM)
After 75-g oral glucose load	30 min	<200 mg/dl (<11.1 mM)
	60 min	<200 mg/dl (<11.1 mM)
	90 min	<200 mg/dl (<11.1 mM)
	120 min	<140 mg/dl (<7.8 mM)

Table 1.4. Indications and Criteria for Screening Tests

INDICATIONS

Screening tests for diabetes mellitus may be indicated when the individual

- has a strong history of diabetes mellitus,
- is markedly obese,
- has a morbid obstetrical history or a history of babies >9 lb at birth,
- is pregnant (between 24 and 28 wk),
- has a history of recurrent skin, genital, or urinary tract infections,
- is > 65 yr,
- has hypertension or hyperlipidemia,
- is of certain races (American Indian, Hispanic, African American), or
- has previously identified IGT.

CRITERIA

Nonpregnant adults: A fasting plasma glucose determination should be used for screening. Fasting plasma glucose level of 115–139 mg/dl (6.4–7.7 mM) is considered an indication for diagnostic testing (Table 1.5). A fasting plasma glucose level >140 mg/dl (>7.8 mM) (if confirmed) meets the criterion for diabetes mellitus.

Pregnant women: An oral glucose challenge (does not have to be fasting) with a 50-g glucose load is recommended for screening. A plasma glucose level ≥140 mg/dl (≥7.8 mM) 1 h later is considered an indication for diagnostic testing.

---

underlying illness, and absence of interfering drugs [Table 1.2]). OGGTs have been used extensively to establish the incidence and prevalence in population-based studies. However, OGGTs may be of limited value in making the diagnosis of diabetes in a given individual due to the intratest variability.

Criteria for the diagnosis of diabetes mellitus and IGT using glucose tolerance tests have been proposed by the National Diabetes Data Group (NDDG) and the World Health Organization (WHO) (Table 1.5). With either criteria, ~20% of OGTTs will yield nondiagnostic values. In the remaining 80%, both classification criteria are equally sensitive.

The OGGT is done using a 75-g oral glucose load. After obtaining a fasting sample, the glucose load is given, and samples are drawn at periodic intervals. A diagnosis of diabetes is made if the venous plasma glucose level is >200 mg/dl (>11.1 mM) at 120 min and one other blood glucose level is also >200 mg/dl (>11.1 mM).

Criteria for Diagnosis of GDM

The criteria for diagnosis of GDM were proposed by O'Sullivan and Mahan in 1964 on the basis of a 100-g OGTT, and they remain unchanged. During normal pregnancy, fasting plasma glucose levels tend to decrease, while post–glucose load levels tend to increase. Thus, criteria for diagnosis of GDM are adjusted appropriately and are calculated to provide maximum sensitivity to diagnose diabetes during pregnancy (Table 1.6). Exceeding two or more of the glucose concentrations noted in Table 1.6 has been demonstrated to cause increased risks to the fetus.

EVALUATION AND CLASSIFICATION OF PATIENTS BEFORE TREATMENT

Before therapy is initiated to treat diabetes mellitus, the patient should have a complete medical evaluation and be classified appropriately.

Table 1.5. Diagnosis of Diabetes Mellitus and Impaired Glucose Tolerance (IGT) by Oral Glucose Tolerance Test (OGTT)

	NDDG criteria		WHO criteria	
	Diabetes mellitus	IGT	Diabetes mellitus	IGT
Fasting	≥140 (7.8)*	<140 (7.8)	≥140 (7.8)	<140 (7.8)
	or	*and*	*or*	*and*
OGTT (2-h glucose)	≥200 (11.1)	140–199 (7.8–11.1)	≥200 (7.8–11.1)	140–199 (7.8–11.1)
OGTT (0.5-h, 1-h, or 1.5-h glucose)	≥200 (11.1)	≥200 (11.1)	(Not part of criteria)	

*mg/dl (mM).
NDDG, National Diabetes Data Group; WHO, World Health Organization.

Evaluation of the Patient

A complete medical evaluation before initiating therapy helps the physician classify the patient, determine the possible presence of underlying diseases that may require further study, and detect the presence of complications frequently associated with diabetes mellitus (see DETECTION AND TREATMENT OF COMPLICATIONS). A reminder list for the evaluation (Table 1.7) is presented on page 10.

Classification of the Patient

The patient should not be classified until all data necessary for making the determination are available. Generally, a reasonably good initial assignment of the patient can be made on the basis of a complete personal and family history and diagnostic test results. The most important distinguishing characteristics of diabetes mellitus and other categories of abnormal glucose intolerance are presented in Table 1.1. Patients should not be classified on the basis of age alone or, in patients whose diabetes was diagnosed after age 40, whether or not they are taking insulin therapy.

There are some special problems in classification that deserve emphasis.

Impaired glucose tolerance. If an individual has a fasting plasma glucose >115 mg/dl (>6.4 mM) but <140 mg/dl (<7.8 mM), he or she has an aproximately equal chance of being nondiabetic, or having IGT or diabetes by the 2-h glucose concentration during an OGTT. These patients are generally classified as having IGT. Because the finding of IGT may identify a person with a higher than normal risk of developing diabetes and atherosclerotic heart disease, these patients should be followed closely. They should be encouraged to achieve and maintain desirable weight and to exercise regularly.

Type I vs. type II diabetes. Another major problem in classification is that it is sometimes difficult to assign the

Table 1.6. Diagnosis of Gestational Diabetes Mellitus (GDM)

After 100-g oral glucose load, diagnosis of GDM may be made if 2 plasma glucose values equal or exceed:

Fasting	105 mg/dl	(5.8 mM)
1 h	190 mg/dl	(10.5 mM)
2 h	165 mg/dl	(9.2 mM)
3 h	145 mg/ld	(8.1 mM)

Table 1.7. Office Guide to Initial Evaluation

Once diagnosis of diabetes mellitus has occurred, the patient should have a complete evaluation, including a search for the presence of complications frequently associated with diabetes. The following is a reminder list for the complete *initial* evaluation.

Medical History

■ Symptoms
■ Results of laboratory tests and special examination results related to the diagnosis of diabetes
■ Prior glycated hemoglobin records
■ Eating patterns, nutritional status, and weight history; growth and development in children and adolescents
■ Details of previous treatment programs, including nutrition and diabetes self-management training
■ Current treatment of diabetes, including medications, meal plan, and results of glucose monitoring and patients' use of data
■ Exercise history
■ Frequency, severity, and cause of acute complications such as ketoacidosis and hypoglycemia
■ Prior or current infections, particularly skin, foot, dental, and genitourinary
■ Symptoms and treatment of chronic complications associated with diabetes
■ Other medications that may affect blood glucose levels
■ Risk factors for atherosclerosis
■ History and treatment of other conditions, including endocrine and eating disorders
■ Family history of diabetes and other endocrine disorders
■ Gestational history

■ Lifestyle, cultural, psychosocial, educational, and economic factors that may influence the management of diabetes.

Physical Examination

■ Height and weight (and comparison to norms in children and adolescents)
■ Sexual maturation (during peripubertal period)
■ Blood pressure determination, including orthostatic measurements when indicated, and comparison to age-related norms
■ Ophthalmoscopic examination, preferably with dilation
■ Oral examination
■ Thyroid palpation
■ Cardiac examination
■ Abdominal examination
■ Evaluation of pulses by palpitation and with auscultation
■ Hand/finger examination
■ Foot examination
■ Skin examination
■ Neurological examination.

Laboratory Evaluation

■ Fasting plasma glucose (a random plasma glucose level may be obtained in an undiagnosed symptomatic patient for diagnostic purposes)
■ Glycated hemoglobin
■ Fasting lipid profile, including total cholesterol, high-density lipoprotein cholesterol, triglycerides, and low-density lipoprotein cholesterol
■ Serum creatinine
■ Urinalysis for glucose, ketones, protein, and evidence of infection
■ Determination for microalbuminuria
■ Urine culture if evidence of infection is present
■ Thyroid function test(s) when indicated

patient to a particular subclass of diabetes mellitus (i.e., type I vs. type II). For example, the thin type II patient who has been taking insulin often looks like a type I patient. Another example is the newly diagnosed child or adolescent who is a member of a family with an autosomal dominant form of inheritance of diabetes (MODY). This patient usually has type II diabetes and should not be classified as having type I diabetes on the basis of age alone. Finally, there are patients with characteristics of type II diabetes who may require insulin therapy for glycemic control but are not dependent on insulin to prevent ketoacidosis or to sustain life. These patients should not be classified as having type I diabetes simply on the basis of their insulin regimen.

It is not necessary for clinicians to determine the presence of islet cell or other antibodies or the degree of insulin secretion. In research studies, the measurement of stimulated plasma C-peptide levels after oral or intravenous stimulus is often used as an index of insulin secretion; however, it has not proved to be a useful classification tool for routine use. In the future, reliable measurements of islet cell or other antibodies may be useful in the classification of diabetes. A history of ketoacidosis or the detection of moderate to strong urine ketones in the presence of hyperglycemia is the most useful indicator of type I diabetes mellitus. Although the classification of some patients may thus be problematic, the goal of therapy remains the achievement of euglycemia.

BIBLIOGRAPHY

Proceedings of the Third International Workshop-Conference on Gestational Diabetes Mellitus. *Diabetes* 40 (Suppl. 2): 1–201, 1991

Harris MI, Hadden WC, Knowler WC, Bennett PH: International criteria for the diagnosis of diabetes and impaired glucose tolerance. *Diabetes Care* 8:562–67, 1985

Keen H: Limitations and problems of diabetes classification from an epidemiological point of view. *Adv Exp Med Biol* 189:31–46, 1985

Little RR, England JD, Wiedmeyer H-M, McKenzie EM, Pettitt DJ, Knowler WC, Goldstein DE: Relationship of glycosylated hemoglobin to oral glucose tolerance. *Diabetes* 37:60–64, 1988

Modan M, Halkin H, Karasik A, Lusky A: Effectiveness of glycated hemoglobin, fasting plasma glucose, and a single post load plasma glucose level in population screening for glucose intolerance. *Am J Epidemiol* 119:431–44, 1984

National Diabetes Data Group: Classification and diagnosis of diabetes mellitus and other categories of glucose intolerance. *Diabetes* 28: 1039–57, 1979

O'Sullivan JB, Mahan CM: Criteria for the oral glucose tolerance test in pregnancy. *Diabetes* 13:278–85, 1964

Roseman JM, Go RCP, Perkins LL, Barger BD, Bell DH, Goldenberg RL, DuBard MB, Huddleston JF, Sedlacek CM, Acton RT: Gestational diabetes mellitus among African-American women. *Diabetes Metab Rev* 7:93–104, 1991

Simon D, Coignet H, Thibult N: Comparison of glycated hemoglobin and fasting plasma glucose with two-hour post-load plasma glucose in the detection of diabetes mellitus. *Am J Epidemiol* 122:589–93, 1985

World Health Organization: *Diabetes mellitus: report of a WHO study group*. Geneva, World Health Org., 1985 (Tech. Rep. Ser., no. 727)

Yudkin JS, Alberti KGMM, McLarty DG, Swai ABM: Impaired glucose tolerance: is it a risk factor for diabetes or a diagnostic ragbag? *Br Med J* 301:397–402, 1990

Pathogenesis

Highlights
Pathogenesis

Non-insulin-dependent (type II) diabetes mellitus is a heterogeneous disorder characterized by diminished tissue (liver, muscle, and adipose tissue) sensitivity to insulin and impaired β-cell function.

In type II diabetes,
- basal insulin concentration is normal or increased;
- insulin secretion in response to intravenous glucose is severely reduced, but responses to other secretagogues are near normal;
- insulin secretion in response to ingested glucose is often impaired but may be normal or increased when viewed in absolute terms; however, relative to the degree of hyperglycemia, insulin secretion is impaired;

- insulin resistance is usually present and may precede diabetes by many years; and
- an initial defect in tissue sensitivity to insulin can lead to the emergence of a defect in insulin secretion: conversely, an impairment in β-cell function can lead to a disturbance in insulin action.

By the time most patients with type II diabetes come to medical attention, significant fasting hyperglycemia is present, and defects in insulin action and insulin secretion are well established. Once the full-blown diabetic syndrome is established, it is impossible to determine in any given individual whether the primary defect originated in the β-cell or in peripheral tissues.

Pathogenesis

INTRODUCTION

Non-insulin-dependent (type II) diabetes mellitus is a heterogeneous disorder characterized by diminished tissue (liver and muscle) sensitivity to insulin impaired β-cell function. There has been considerable debate as to which defect (i.e., impaired insulin secretion or impaired insulin action) is the initial lesion in the pathogenesis of type II diabetes. It is clear, however, that both insulin secretion and insulin action are markedly impaired in diabetic individuals who have had the disease for any significant length of time and who have moderately severe fasting hyperglycemia (plasma glucose >180–200 mg/dl [>10.0–11.1 mM]).

In recent years, a significant body of evidence has accumulated that indicates that defects in insulin secretion can lead to insulin resistance and vice versa. Thus, once the full-blown diabetic syndrome has become established, it is impossible to determine in any given individual whether the primary defect originated in the β-cell or in peripheral/hepatic tissues.

Obviously, more information about the relationship between abnormalities in insulin secretion and insulin action is needed for a full understanding of type II diabetes. Nonetheless, certain general statements about the pathogenesis of type II diabetes can be made.

INSULIN SECRETION

In nondiabetic individuals, there are two phases of insulin release: *1)* an early phase that occurs within the first few minutes after intravenous glucose injection and that represents the release of insulin stored within the β-cell and *2)* a later phase of insulin secretion that includes newly synthesized insulin. The relative contribution of these two phases to insulin secretion that occurs after oral glucose ingestion is not known.

Fasting Insulin Concentration

Patients with type II diabetes mellitus usually have normal or elevated fasting plasma insulin levels. This postabsorptive hyperinsulinemia reflects an augmented basal rate of insulin secretion that occurs in response to insulin resistance and/or elevated fasting plasma glucose concentrations. The fasting insulin level is diminished only when marked fasting hyperglycemia (>250–300 mg/dl [>13.9–16.7 mM]) occurs. When this happens, β-cell function is severely disturbed.

Glucose-Stimulated Insulin Response

In individuals with impaired glucose tolerance and fasting plasma glucose levels <115 mg/dl (<16.4 mM), the total plasma insulin response after oral or intravenous glucose administration is normal or, more often, elevated. When the fasting plasma glucose concentration exceeds 115 mg/dl (>6.4 mM) in an individual with impaired glucose tolerance, the rapid release of insulin after food ingestion usually is decreased; however, the later release of insulin may be equal to or greater than normal.

In diabetic patients with moderate fasting hyperglycemia (140–180 mg/dl [7.8–10.0 mM]), the rapid release of insulin is further decreased as is the late phase of insulin secretion. Because these individuals are markedly insulin resistant (see subsequent discussion), even a "normal" plasma insulin response is, in fact, abnormal and inadequate to maintain normal glucose tolerance. In nondiabetic individuals, the presence of insulin resistance (such as in obesity) is compensated for by an increase in insulin secretion. As the diabetic state progressively worsens and more severe fasting hyperglycemia (>180–200 mg/dl [>10.0–11.1 mM]) ensues, the plasma insulin response to both intravenous and oral glucose becomes progressively diminished. Overall, inadequate insulin secretory response to glucose is a hallmark of type II diabetes. The molecular mechanism of this impairment is not known for the vast majority of patients. The diagnostic criteria for impaired glucose tolerance and for diabetes mellitus

15

are presented in DIAGNOSIS AND CLASSI-FICATION OF DIABETES MELLITUS, Table 1.5 (page 9).

Physiologic Consequences of Impaired Insulin Secretion

The impairment in insulin secretion has important physiologic consequences. When the early phase of insulin release is reduced, the portal vein insulin concentration remains low after food ingestion and hepatic glucose production is not suppressed. Continued output of glucose by the liver, supplemented by glucose entering the circulation via the gastrointestinal tract, leads to excessive hyperglycemia. In addition, glucose uptake by peripheral tissues is not appropriate for the prevailing glucose and insulin concentrations. Early in the pathogenesis of diabetes, this leads to enhanced secretion of insulin during the hours after glucose ingestion. In these individuals, plasma glucose concentration will return to normal but only at the expense of the resultant late hyperglycemia and hyperinsulinemia. As the defect in β-cell secretion becomes more severe, the late phase of insulin secretion is diminished. When this happens, fasting hyperglycemia and frank diabetes develop. The severity of the glucose intolerance following food ingestion closely parallels the defect in insulin secretion.

Summary

In type II diabetes mellitus, β-cell function is impaired, but in response to insulin resistance and fasting hyperglycemia, basal insulin concentration is normal or increased. In individuals with impaired glucose tolerance, the total plasma insulin response to a glucose challenge is usually increased, even though the early insulin response is decreased. In patients with type II diabetes and moderate to severe fasting hyperglycemia (>180–200 mg/dl [>10.0–11.1 mM]), all phases of insulin secretion are markedly impaired. With intermediate fasting plasma glucose levels (120–180 mg/dl [6.7–10.0 mM]),

the plasma insulin response to glucose may be increased, normal, or decreased and, in general, is inversely correlated with the degree of fasting hyperglycemia. However, insulin responses are inappropriately low relative to the prevailing plasma glucose concentration.

INSULIN RESISTANCE

Insulin resistance is an early defect and is present in the majority of individuals with impaired glucose tolerance and essentially in all patients with type II diabetes mellitus who have fasting plasma glucose levels ≥140 mg/dl (>7.8 mM). Insulin resistance also is commonly present in nondiabetic relatives of individuals with type II diabetes mellitus. An impairment in endogenous insulin action was first suggested by the observation that many patients with type II diabetes have normal or increased plasma insulin responses after glucose ingestion. Subsequently, numerous investigators, with a variety of different experimental techniques, have demonstrated the presence of insulin resistance in most patients with type II diabetes. The insulin resistance is positively correlated with the elevation in fasting plasma glucose concentration. Thus, individuals with greater glucose intolerance are more insulin resistant than those with lesser degrees of glucose intolerance.

Sites of Insulin Resistance

Numerous studies demonstrate that insulin resistance exists in both hepatic and peripheral tissues. Although this discussion focuses on the consequences of insulin resistance on glucose metabolism, it should be acknowledged that insulin has important effects on a variety of other metabolic processes, abnormalities of which may have important consequences, particularly in the development of the complications of diabetes. Impairment in muscle glucose uptake is accompanied by impaired nonoxidative pathways of glucose utilization, primarily glycogen formation, as well as a slight decrease in glucose oxidation. The decrease in insulin-mediated muscle glucose disposal contributes to the excessive rise in plasma glucose concentration after glucose ingestion.

Despite the presence of fasting hyperinsulinemia, basal rates of hepatic glucose production are almost invariably increased when the fasting plasma glucose concentration exceeds 140 mg/dl (>7.8 mM). Furthermore, the increase in basal hepatic glucose production is correlated with the level of fasting plasma glucose. When insulin is infused at a low concentration, patients with type II diabetes fail to demonstrate a normal suppression of hepatic glucose output, indicating the presence of hepatic insulin resistance. However, at high infusion rates, hepatic glucose output is suppressed by insulin.

Mechanisms of Insulin Resistance at Cellular Level

In the most general sense, the action of insulin involves two processes. First, insulin binds to a specific receptor located on the cell surface. Second, this interaction activates a series of intracellular events, culminating in enhanced glucose transport and stimulation of a variety of intracellular enzymatic pathways. For the sake of simplicity, all the intracellular processes involved in insulin action after it binds to its receptor will be referred to as postbinding events.

Binding Abnormalities

Insulin binding to its specific cell surface receptor is the first stage in the mechanism of insulin action. Therefore, reduction in insulin binding would result in impaired insulin action. This situation may be found in patients with mutations in the insulin gene or insulin receptor gene. However, these abnormalities account for <1% of patients with type II diabetes. Because most patients with type II diabetes mellitus are obese and hyperinsulinemic, this decreased binding may be secondary to obesity and/or hyperinsulinemia. Studies on liver, muscle, and adipose tissue have also demonstrated reduced insulin binding. Thus, a decrease

in insulin binding is unlikely to play a role in the insulin resistance of the common forms of type II diabetes.

Postbinding Abnormalities

Postbinding abnormalities are primarily responsible for the insulin resistance in patients with type II diabetes who have significant fasting hyperglycemia. These defects include a marked decrease in glucose transport and other intracellular processes involved in glucose metabolism, especially insulin-stimulated glycogen synthesis.

Insulin-mediated glucose transport is facilitated by a specific insulin-regulatable glucose transporter (GLUT-4), which is present in muscle and adipocytes. Yet, abnormalities in GLUT-4 have not been found to be responsible for the insulin resistance seen in most patients with type II diabetes. Several families with a molecular defect in the hexokinase gene have been described. These patients manifest maturity-onset diabetes of the young, an uncommon form of type II diabetes.

Several intracellular steps of insulin action have been identified. Impairment at any given level of signal transduction may result in inappropriate insulin action, i.e., insulin resistance. With the identification of these intracellular steps, the search for the defect(s) responsible for type II diabetes has intensified.

Summary

In patients with type II diabetes, postbinding abnormalities are primarily responsible for the insulin resistance. Impaired insulin binding when present may be secondary to associated obesity and hyperinsulinemia but, nevertheless, may also contribute to impaired tissue insulin sensitivity.

PATHOGENETIC SEQUENCES LEADING TO TYPE II DIABETES MELLITUS

By the time most patients with type II diabetes mellitus come to medical attention, significant fasting hyperglycemia

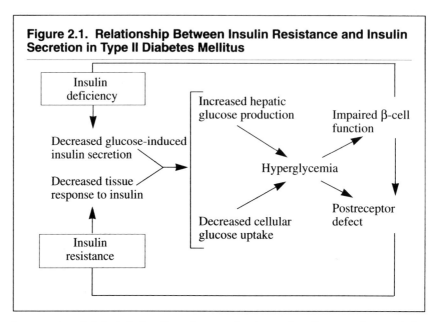

Figure 2.1. Relationship Between Insulin Resistance and Insulin Secretion in Type II Diabetes Mellitus

is present, and defects in insulin action and insulin secretion are well established. With current knowledge, it is difficult to know which defect occurred first in the natural history of the disease. What seems to be evolving as a common theme is that abnormalities in insulin secretion can lead to the development of insulin resistance, and conversely, an impairment in glucose uptake by peripheral tissues may secondarily eventuate in β-cell failure. The interrelationship between the two principal mechanisms (i.e., impaired insulin secretion and insulin resistance) responsible for glucose intolerance in type II diabetes is presented in Figure 2.1.

In essentially all patients with type II diabetes, the insulin secretory response to glucose is delayed, and in many it is absolutely diminished (Figure 2.1). In addition, the pulsatile pattern of secretion commonly observed in nondiabetic individuals is either absent or diminished in people with type II diabetes. This defective insulin secretory response leads to inadequate suppression of hepatic glucose production and a decrease in glucose uptake by peripheral tissues during the period immediately after glucose ingestion. The resulting postprandial hyperglycemia provides a persistent stimulus to insulin secretion, and the resultant hyperinsulinemia will eventually return the plasma glucose concentration to normal. However, fasting euglycemia will be maintained only at the expense of an increased plasma insulin concentration.

Insulin is an important factor involved in the regulation of its own receptor. Thus, chronic hyperinsulinemia will cause a downregulation of the number of insulin receptors. Chronic hyperinsulinemia may also lead to postbinding defects. Both of these mechanisms can lead to the development of insulin resistance. The clinical counterpart of this pathogenetic sequence is a patient with impaired glucose tolerance. This individual is characterized by a decreased early plasma insulin response to glucose, a normal or increased total plasma insulin response, reduced insulin binding, impaired suppression of hepatic glucose production, and reduced peripheral glucose uptake. Postbinding alterations in glucose utilization may be present.

As the insulin response to glucose becomes progressively more deficient, fasting hyperglycemia occurs. The progressive nature of the insulin secretory abnormality may result from several factors: *1)* the natural history of the β-cell defect, which may be genetically determined; *2)* persistent hyperglycemia, which can have detrimental effects on the β-cell and can cause a progressive impairment in insulin secretion; or *3)* some other, as yet unrecognized, metabolic disturbance that is present in the diabetic milieu.

As β-cell function becomes progressively impaired, the insulin secretory response becomes deficient, hyperglycemia occurs, and a postbinding defect in insulin action becomes more evident. In the basal state, the majority (~70%) of glucose is taken up by insulin-independent tissues, primarily brain, and therefore, the major factor responsible for fasting hyperglycemia is increased hepatic glucose production. After glucose ingestion, insulin-dependent tissues (primarily muscle and liver) become more important in the disposal of a glucose load. Thus, when the β-cell response becomes absolutely diminished, marked postbinding abnormalities (i.e., glucose transport and intracellular glucose metabolism) develop. The development of fasting hyperglycemia further aggravates the insulin resistance.

The clinical picture that emerges from the sequence of events just described is typical of the patient with type II diabetes. Both the early and late phases of insulin secretion are impaired, and marked peripheral tissue (muscle) insulin resistance is present. Although some patients may have diminished insulin binding, postbinding abnormalities are primarily responsible for the defect in insulin action. Such individuals with type II diabetes have elevated rates of hepatic glucose production both before and after eating. The ability of insulin to suppress hepatic glucose output and increase glucose utilization is also impaired.

CONCLUSION

In summary, both tissue sensitivity to insulin and β-cell secretion are in a dynamic state of flux in type II diabetes mellitus. Insulin resistance can lead to the development of a defect in insulin secretion, and, similarly, impaired β-cell function can lead to a disturbance in insulin action. This explains why both insulin resistance and impaired insulin secretion are so uniformly observed in type II diabetes once the full-blown diabetic syndrome is established.

BIBLIOGRAPHY

Campbell PJ, Mandarino LJ, Gerich J: Quantification of the relative impairments in actions of insulin on hepatic glucose production and peripheral glucose uptake in NIDDM. *Metabolism* 32:151–56, 1988

Moller DE, Flier JS: Insulin resistance mechanisms, syndromes, and implications. *N Engl J Med* 325:938–48, 1991

Dinneen S, Gerich J, Rizza RA: Carbohydrate metabolism in non-insulin-dependent diabetes mellitus. *N Engl J Med* 327:707–13, 1992

DeFronzo RA, Bonadonna RC, Ferrannini E: Pathogenesis of NIDDM: a balanced overview. *Diabetes Care* 15:318–68, 1992

Management

Highlights

Therapeutic Objectives and Plan
Introduction

Nutrition
Introduction
Body Weight
Protein
Carbohydrate and Fat
Alternative Sweeteners and Fat Substitutes
Vitamins/Minerals
Alcohol

Exercise
Introduction
Potential Benefits of Exercise
Precautions and Considerations
The Exercise Prescription

Pharmacologic Intervention
Introduction
Treatment With Oral Hypoglycemic Agents
Insulin Therapy
Combination Therapy: Insulin Plus Oral Agent
Adverse Drug Reactions

Special Therapeutic Problems
Introduction
Pregnancy
Surgery

Assessment of Treatment Efficacy
Introduction
Office Methods
Self-Monitoring

Highlights
Management

THERAPEUTIC OBJECTIVES AND PLAN

The two major management goals of type II diabetes mellitus are to
■ achieve normal metabolic biochemical control, and
■ prevent microvascular and macrovascular complications.

Specific goals of therapy are to
■ eliminate symptoms,
■ optimize metabolic parameters,
■ assist the patient to achieve and maintain desirable body weight,
■ improve cardiovascular risk factors, and
■ prevent and treat microvascular complications.

Recommended treatment modalities include
■ dietary modification,
■ regular physical activity, and
■ pharmacologic intervention with either an oral hypoglycemic agent or insulin.

Individualize therapy based on patient age, other illnesses, lifestyle, financial restrictions, self-management skills learned, and level of patient motivation.

Recommendations for glycemic control are found in Table 3.1

Patient education that enhances self-care behaviors is essential for the successful management of type II diabetes mellitus.

NUTRITION

Medical nutrition therapy is the most important element in the therapeutic plan for patients with type II diabetes. For some, nutrition and exercise are the only interventions needed to control the metabolic abnormalities associated with type II diabetes, including hyperglycemia, hyperlipidemia, and hypertension.

When the person with diabetes is overweight, total caloric intake should be decreased to produce a lasting weight loss. Caloric restriction itself is usually successful in lowering plasma glucose levels even before substantial weight loss is achieved. Approaches to weight reduction are outlined on pages 30–31.

Patients with type II diabetes who are of normal weight should eat sufficient calories to maintain that weight and should distribute calories/carbohydrate intake throughout the day to optimize blood glucose control.

Recommendations for nutrient content of the diet, including fat, protein, carbohydrates, and micronutrients, are presented on page 29.

Patients with diabetes have greater-than-normal prevalence of hyperlipidemia, atherosclerosis, and hypertension. Nutrition recommendations should consider these conditions yet be individualized.

The use of alcohol and sweeteners is discussed on pages 33–34.

Successful implementation of a specific nutrition plan requires
■ patient education and behavior modification,
■ individualization of the meal plan, and
■ continuous follow-up.

Early intervention and follow up with a dietitian greatly facilitates successful nutrition management.

22

EXERCISE

Unless contraindicated, appropriate physical activity is strongly recommended to maximize the effects of dietary modification.

The potential benefits of increased physical activity include
- improvement in insulin sensitivity and improvement in glucose tolerance,
- promotion of weight loss and maintenance of desirable body weight when combined with restricted caloric intake,
- improvement of cardiovascular risk factors,
- potential reduction in dosage or need for insulin or oral hypoglycemic agents,
- enhancement of work capacity, and
- enrichment of quality of life and improvement in sense of well-being.

In some patients requiring hypo-glycemic medication, potential hazards are associated with increased physical activity, including hypoglycemia during or after exercise.

Exercise should be prescribed with caution if the patient has poorly controlled, labile blood glucose levels or is at increased risk because of microvascular and/or cardiovascular complications.

PHARMACOLOGIC INTERVENTION

When the patient has been adequately trained and trialed on diet/exercise and continues to fail to achieve normal or near-normal plasma glucose levels, pharmacologic intervention should be considered.

Pharmacologic intervention is an adjunct to and not a substitute for dietary modification and exercise.

The choice between oral hypoglycemic agent and insulin should be made with the particular patient in mind, taking into account
- the level of blood glucose control desired,
- the total clinical context of the patient's disease,
- the patient's acceptance of the various therapeutic modalities,
- the patient's age and weight,
- the patient's ability for self-care management,
- the patient's level of diabetes education, and
- the patient's level of motivation.

One group of oral hypoglycemic agents (sulfonylureas) augments β-cell insulin secretion acutely. After several months, insulin levels return to pretreatment values, whereas glucose levels remain improved, which suggests that sulfonylurea agents exert pancreatic and extrapancreatic effects on glucose metabolism.

Oral hypoglycemic agents differ from one another in terms of potency, pharmacokinetics, and metabolism (Table 3.7).

Approximately 70% of patients with type II diabetes demonstrate an initial satisfactory response to sulfonylurea therapy.

The patient who is most likely to respond to oral agents
- has had onset of diabetes after 40 yr of age,
- has had diabetes for <5 yr, and
- has never received insulin or has been well controlled on <40 U/day.

About 5–10% of patients each year experience secondary failure, which may be due to failure of the patient to follow the prescribed dietary plan, progression of disease, or the occur-rence of an underlying stressful disease or condition.

Oral hypoglycemic agents are con-traindicated if the patient
- has type I diabetes,
- is pregnant or lactating,

■ has a stressful concurrent condition with significant hyperglycemia, or
■ is allergic to sulfa drugs.

Side effects of sulfonylureas are relatively uncommon. The principal adverse reaction to sulfonylurea therapy is hypoglycemia. Elderly patients are more susceptible to hypoglycemia induced by oral agents, particularly when they skip meals and when hepatic, renal, or cardiovascular function is impaired. In these individuals, longer-acting sulfonylureas should be used with caution.

The iminent introduction of the biguanide metformin will give the clinician another oral hypoglycemic agent in the therapeutic armamentarium. Because metformin does not increase insulin secretion, it may represent a good choice as additional or adjunctive therapy to sulfonylureas,

Factors that influence the choice of oral hypoglycemic agent are outlined on page 43. When prescribing an oral agent initially, the lowest effective dose should be used, and the dose should be increased every 1 or 2 wk until desired glycemic control is achieved or until the maximum dose is reached. Some patients maintained on low doses of oral hypoglycemic agents can discontinue the agents and control glucose levels with nutrition and exercise.

It is possible for insulin to achieve satisfactory blood glucose control in patients with type II diabetes. However, insulin resistance—particularly in those who are obese—may be difficult to overcome and may require large quantities of insulin.

Several circumstances demand the use of insulin in type II diabetic patients, such as
■ periods of acute injury, infection, or surgery;
■ pregnancy; or
■ allergy or serious reaction to sulfonylurea agents.

Human insulin is indicated for patients with insulin allergy, severe insulin resistance due to insulin antibodies, lipoatrophy, onset of diabetes during pregnancy, or acute problems that require intermittent insulin therapy.

The insulin prescription depends on the desired course of action. Some patients with mild to moderate fasting hyperglycemia may be adequately controlled with one injection of intermediate-acting insulin before breakfast or at bedtime. Many patients require a multidose regimen consisting of short-acting insulin in combination with either intermediate-acting or long-acting insulin (Figure 3.1).

The complications of insulin therapy include hypoglycemia, lipodystrophies, antibody formation including insulin resistance, and allergy (both local and systemic). Some of these complications are minimized by the use of human insulin.

In select patients who have failed to achieve control on oral agents, an injection of intermediate-acting insulin at night has been used in combination with morning administration of a sulfonylurea.

Several drugs in common use today can cause hyperglycemia or hypoglycemia (Table 3.8). When possible, these drugs should be avoided.

SPECIAL THERAPEUTIC PROBLEMS: PREGNANCY AND SURGERY

Ideally, pregnancy in a patient with diabetes should be planned so that conception occurs when the patient has normal fasting, preprandial, and postprandial plasma glucose levels. Patients should obtain preconception counseling from the health-care team. Referral should be considered if the plasma glucose level >120 mg/dl (6.7 mM) at any time during pregnancy.

The major principles governing the management of diabetes during surgery are presented in Table 3.12. The objectives of management before, during, and after surgery are to prevent hypoglycemia and hyperglycemia.

ASSESSMENT OF TREATMENT EFFICACY

The therapeutic response to treatment of diabetes mellitus is monitored by determining effects on glucose and lipid metabolism. Physicians monitor the responses to treatment with determinations of fasting, preprandial, and postprandial plasma glucose levels (an index of day-to-day control) and with assays for glycated hemoglobin (a reflection of degree of glucose control for the preceding 2–3 mo).

Patients can determine the effects of therapy by self-monitoring of blood glucose (SMBG) and measurement of urine ketones when necessary. They can use a daily journal to record food intake, exercise, doses of insulin or oral hypoglycemic agent, symptoms, and results of self-administered blood tests.

Problem solving with SMBG makes it possible for many patients to achieve euglycemia.

Therapeutic Objectives and Plan

INTRODUCTION

There are two major management goals for the patient with type II diabetes: *1)* to achieve normal metabolic control, and *2)* to prevent microvascular and macrovascular complications. To achieve the first goal, the physician adjusts elements of the treatment plan to produce normal levels of fasting and postprandial plasma glucose, fasting low-density lipoprotein (LDL) and high-density lipoprotein (HDL) cholesterol and triglycerides, and glycated hemoglobin. To prevent or delay the onset of microvascular and neuropathic complications of diabetes, it is important to normalize blood glucose levels. To prevent or delay macrovascular complications, it is also important to normalize lipid levels, lower elevated blood pressure to normal, and help the patient to stop smoking and approach desirable body weight.

There is evidence that long-term glycemic control can prevent or ameliorate the microvascular and neuropathic complications of diabetes. The Diabetes Control and Complications Trial (DCCT) demonstrated definitively the beneficial and slowing progression of retinopathy, nephropathy, and neuropathy in type I diabetes. Although no intervention trial in type II diabetes has demonstrated a beneficial impact of intensive treatment regimens on complications, it is reasonable to extrapolate the beneficial effects noted in the DCCT to type II diabetes. The accelerated atherosclerosis seen in patients with type II diabetes may also be ameliorated with normalization of plasma glucose levels over the long term.

A rational approach to the treatment of patients with type II diabetes should include measures that will specifically reverse the underlying pathogenic metabolic disturbances that result in hyperglycemia, i.e., insulin resistance and impaired β-cell function. Various approaches may be used. First, it is critical to educate the patient and his/her family on self-care practices necessary to manage diabetes. National standards exist for diabetes education programs, and these should be followed. In addition, a meal plan and exercise program should be developed. Pharmacologic therapy should be instituted if necessary. An approach should be developed to make continuous assessment of metabolic control. Within this scheme, careful attention to psychosocial influences and/or behavior-modification techniques are exceptionally valuable. Finally, the physician must have indices that indicate results of attempts at glycemic control (Table 3.1). Although it is recognized that normal glucose levels may not always be achieved, this remains the goal of optimal therapy. Of course, plasma glucose goals should not be achieved at the expense of recurrent episodes of severe hypoglycemia.

If members of the health-care team accept these management goals; follow

Table 3.1. Glycemic Control			
BIOCHEMICAL INDEX	**NORMAL**	**GOAL**	**ACTION SUGGESTED**
Fasting/preprandial glucose	<115 mg/dl (<6.4 mM)	<120 mg/dl (<6.7 mM)	<80 or >140 mg/dl (<4.4 or >7.8 mM)
Bedtime glucose	<120 mg/dl (<6.7 mM)	100–140 mg/dl (5.6–7.8 mM)	<100 or >160 mg/dl (<5.6 or >8.9 mM)
Glycated hemoglobin*	<6%	<7%	>8%

*Referenced to a nondiabetic range of 4–6% (mean 5%, SD 0.5%).

suggested approaches; use the indices of glycemic management; and strive to correct the vascular risk factors of obesity, dyslipidemia, hypertension, and cigarette smoking, they will help their patients with type II diabetes improve their lifestyle and prevent or delay vascular complications.

BIBLIOGRAPHY

American Diabetes Association position statement: Standards of medical care for patients with diabetes mellitus. *Diabetes Care* 17:616–24, 1994

DeFronzo RA, Ferrannini E, Koivisto V: New concepts in the pathogenesis and treatment of noninsulin dependent diabetes mellitus. *Am J Med* 74:5281, 1983

Gordon T, Castelli WP, Hjortland MC, Kannel WB, Dawber, TR: Diabetes, blood lipids and the role of obesity in CHD risk for women: the Framingham study. *Ann Intern Med* 87:393–97, 1977.

Nutrition

INTRODUCTION

Medical nutrition therapy is the most important element in the therapeutic plan for individuals with type II diabetes. In fact, for many people with mild to moderate diabetes, an appropriate combination of nutrition and exercise is the only therapeutic intervention needed to effectively control the metabolic abnormalities associated with this disease. The goals of nutrition therapy in type II diabetes are

- maintaining near-normal blood glucose levels,
- normalizing serum lipid levels,
- attaining and maintaining a reasonable body weight, and
- promoting overall health.

Due to the heterogeneous nature of type II diabetes, there is no single prescription for dietary modification that will achieve these goals in all patients. The meal plan must be individualized. Diversity in insulin secretion capacity and insulin resistance, as well as personal characteristics related to lifestyle, age, body weight, and medication regimen, influence strategies chosen to achieve the nutrition goals. Because type II diabetes occurs primarily in adults, eating habits, attitude, and learning abilities also influence the ability to achieve these goals. Guidelines for the nutritional management of individuals with diabetes have been developed that consider the heterogeneity of diabetes (Table 3.2). The guidelines emphasize that nutrition intervention should be based on a thorough assessment of each person's usual and customary intake and nutritional status and that intervention need not be dramatic to have an impact. Furthermore, intervention is ongoing throughout the life span and should be outcome driven. The success of a particular dietary intervention is evaluated via metabolic parameters, e.g., self-monitoring of blood glucose (SMBG) results, glycated hemoglobin, and serum lipids. Failure of one intervention strategy does not preclude using another.

BODY WEIGHT

Calories/Distribution

Because body weight profoundly influences insulin resistance, insulin requirements, and blood glucose control, an appropriate caloric intake is a key component of the nutrition plan in type II diabetes. Average/usual daily calorie intake can be evaluated with a 24-h diet recall or a 3-day history. This assessment can also identify fat, carbohydrate, and protein intake and distribution of these nutrients between meals and snacks.

Normal Weight

About 10–20% of people with type II diabetes are within their normal weight range and, therefore, may not need their caloric intake modified. Occasionally, they may be underweight and need caloric intake increased. Because most normal- weight individuals can internally/automatically monitor their food intake, other dietary modifications such as shifting calories between meals, particularly carbohydrate calories, may be the primary dietary modification. Many individuals, for example, cannot tolerate large amounts of calories and carbohydrate in the morning.

The distribution of calories and carbohydrate between meals and snacks should be driven by the level of glucose control desired. There is no set pattern, and equal distribution has not proved necessary for improved metabolic control. SMBG results are used to guide such decisions. People taking insulin can adjust their dosage to calorie/carbohydrate amounts by evaluating 2-h postprandial glucose levels. Those taking oral agents or on nutrition therapy alone often need to allow 4–5 h between meals. This schedule accommodates the sluggish rate of pancreatic insulin secretion common in type II diabetes. Some individuals, particularly those on oral agents, may require or desire between-meal snacks to help control hunger or moderate blood glucose levels.

Table 3.2. Nutrition Goals, Principles, and Recommendations

Calories
■ Sufficient to attain and/or maintain a reasonable body weight for adults, normal growth and development for children and adolescents, and adequate nutrition during pregnancy and lactation

Protein
■ 10–20% of daily calories
■ No less than adult RDA ($0.8 \text{ g}^{-1}\cdot\text{kg}\cdot\text{day}^{-1}$) with evidence of nephropathy

Fat
■ Saturated fat <10% of daily calories, <7% with elevated LDL
■ Polyunsaturated fat up to 10% of total calories
■ Remaining total fat varies with treatment goals
  ■ ~30%—normal weight and lipids
  ■ <30%—obese, elevated LDL
  ■ <40%—elevated triglycerides unresponsive to fat restriction and weight loss
  ■ Predominately monounsaturated fat

Cholesterol
■ <300 mg/day

Carbohydrate
■ Difference after protein and fat goals have been met
■ Percentage varies with treatment goals

Sweeteners
■ Sucrose need not be restricted, must be substituted as carbohydrate
■ Nutritive sweeteners have no advantage over sucrose, must be substituted as carbohydrate
■ Nonnutritive sweeteners approved by the FDA are safe to consume

Fiber
■ 20–35 g/day, same as general population

Sodium
■ <3000 mg/day
■ <2400 mg/day in mild to moderate hypertension

Alcohol
■ Moderate usage, i.e., <2 alcoholic beverages daily

Vitamins/Minerals
■ Same as general population
■ Magnesium replacement possibly needed if at high risk

Goals must always be individualized. RDA, recommended dietary allowance; LDL, low-density lipoprotein.
Adapted from American Diabetes Association position statement: Nutrition recommendations: see Bibliography

Overweight

Approximately 80–90% of people with type II diabetes are obese, thus weight loss is usually the primary treatment goal. Calorie restriction itself may be responsible for improved glucose tolerance, because the loss of as little as

Table 3.3. Suggested Weight for Adults

HEIGHT*	WEIGHT (lb)†	
	19–34 yr	≥35 yr
5'0"	97–128	108–138
5'1"	101–132	111–143
5'2"	104–137	115–148
5'3"	107–141	119–152
5'4"	111–146	122–157
5'5"	114–150	126–162
5'6"	118–155	130–167
5'7"	121–160	134–172
5'8"	125–164	138–178
5'9"	129–169	142–183
5'10"	132–174	146–188
5'11"	136–179	151–194
6'0"	140–184	155–199
6'1"	144–189	159–205
6'2"	148–195	164–210
6'3"	152–200	168–216
6'4"	156–205	173–222
6'5"	160–211	173–222
6'6"	164–216	182–234

From The Dietary Guidelines for Americans, U.S. Department of Agriculture, U.S. Department of Health and Human Services, 3rd ed., 1990
*Without shoes. †Without clothes.

5–10% of body weight improves glucose uptake, reduces insulin secretion, and decreases hepatic glucose production. Weight loss may be most beneficial early in the diagnosis of type II diabetes when insulin secretion is greatest. In fact, weight reduction and exercise are the therapeutic regimens most useful for people with impaired glucose tolerance.

Weight reduction may be accomplished by a combination of modest caloric restriction, exercise, behavior modification of eating habits, and psychosocial support. Although most clinicians agree on this, many seriously overweight individuals find weight loss and, more important, weight maintenance difficult. Genetic predisposition to obesity and possible impaired metabolic and appetite regulation may influence a person's ability to lose weight via any regimen. Furthermore, most individuals will regain lost weight. Such fluctuations in weight have been shown to be detrimental to health in modestly overweight individuals. It remains to be seen if severely overweight individuals (body mass index [BMI; kg/m^2] >30) are similarly affected by such fluctuations.

BMI is the most frequently used expression of body fatness. It does not take into account distribution of body fat, muscle mass, or age. Generally, body fatness increases slightly with age, although debate exists over whether this is an effect of aging or decreased muscle mass from lack of exercise. Body fat distributed above the waist increases the risk of developing diabetes, cardiovascular disease, and hypertension. Fortunately, body fat stored above the waist is easier to lose than fat stored below the waist.

Because of the psychological and physiological impact of "dieting," obese individuals should be encouraged to attain a reasonable body weight (Table 3.3). The higher weights in the ranges in Table 3.3 generally apply to men, who tend to have more muscle and bone; the lower weights more often apply to women, who have less muscle and bone. Note that reasonable weight is defined as the weight an individual and health-care provider acknowledge as achievable and maintainable, both short and long term. This may not be the same as traditionally defined desirable or ideal body weight.

A 3500-cal deficit will produce a loss of 1 lb of body fat. Daily calorie intake should be evaluated with a diet history and adjusted to produce a deficit. Generally, a decrease of 500–1000 cal/day is needed to produce a 1- to 2-lb loss of fat per week. This can vary, however, based on the individual and his/her willingness to restrict intake and/or increase activity. Regular exercise enhances weight loss in dieting individuals and is identified as a predictor for successful weight maintenance. Because a restriction of <1200 cal for women and <1500 cal for men is difficult to adhere to and can be nutritionally inadequate, some individuals may do better by reducing daily intake by 250 cal and increasing daily activity by 250 cal. If the diet history is unreliable, as may be the case in obese individuals, approximate daily calorie intake can be estimated by multiplying actual weight by a factor of 10–15 (factor decreases with age).

Alternative approaches for calorie restriction are possible with individuals who are seriously overweight. Very restrictive low-calorie diets (600–800 cal/day) are sometimes used in type II diabetes. This medically supervised approach generally involves a liquid formula but may be accomplished with high-quality lean-protein sources (1.5 g · kg^{-1} · day^{-1}) with vitamin and mineral supplementation. Weight loss is rapid (3–5 lb/wk), and hyperglycemia generally improves within 24 h of implementation. Near-maximum blood glucose improvement is achieved within 10 days of initiating this regimen. However, this approach should be restricted to individuals who are at least 30% above desirable weight (BMI >30). For some, using this regimen for as short a period as 2–12 wk can provide the psychological motivation needed to encourage dietary adherence and may, in fact, delay or prevent the necessity for pharmacologic therapy. Alternating a very-low-calorie dietary regimen with a modest caloric reduction has been used successfully in some studies and may be a potential alternative for certain individuals.

Nonaddictive appetite suppressants may be useful for some patients with type II diabetes. Also, studies with serotonin inhibitors (e.g., phentermine and fenfluramine) in combination with appetite suppressants have yielded promising results. Most people will regain the lost weight once the suppressant is stopped. Therefore, research into the potential long-term use of these drugs is ongoing.

People with type II diabetes who take oral hypoglycemic agents or insulin will require a decrease in drug dosage or discontinuation of the drug as weight loss progresses. This may be a gradual reduction with a modestly hypocaloric diet or a rapid reduction (50%) with a very-low-calorie diet. Failure to decrease the doses of these drugs can compromise weight-loss efforts because hypoglycemia and its treatment increase calorie intake. In addition, some research and considerable anecdotal evidence suggest that excessive insulin therapy may also lead to hunger and overeating, which is counterproductive in obesity.

SMBG provides the necessary feedback to make adjustments in nutrition therapy. Frequent follow-up with a dietitian provides the problem-solving techniques, encouragement, and support the weight-loss efforts require. This can be done individually or in groups. Appropriate referrals to local hospital programs or other weight-loss programs with qualified staff are useful.

PROTEIN

The recommendation for protein intake in type II diabetes is the U.S. recommended dietary allowance (RDA) of 0.8 g · kg^{-1} · day^{-1} for adults. Typically, larger amounts are consumed in Western diets (1.2–2.0 g · kg^{-1} · day^{-1}). Thus, protein accounts for ~12–20% or more of total calorie consumption. Because excessive protein consumption may aggravate renal insufficiency, 0.8–1.0 g · kg^{-1} · day^{-1} may represent an optimal goal in type II diabetes. This goal should be accomplished gradually over several months or years, because it represents a major alteration in attitude toward protein in the diet. Meat, fish, and poultry would be limited to 3–5 oz/day on such a regimen. More severe restriction (0.6 g · kg^{-1} · day^{-1}) has been suggested to reduce proteinuria and slow the progression of renal failure in patients who exhibit some renal insufficiency. Compliance with such a regimen is difficult, and studies have suggested muscle wasting and loss of total-body protein can result. Therefore, individuals with diabetes should not consume <0.8 g · kg^{-1} · day^{-1} of protein. Increasing evidence suggests that vegetable protein is not nephrotoxic and need not be restricted. There is limited evidence that individuals with type II diabetes continue to secrete insulin in response to protein ingestion. The glycemic effect of adding or subtracting protein from a given meal or snack can be evaluated with SMBG.

Table 3.4. Fatty Acid Composition of Selected Fats (Percentage of Total Lipid)*

TYPE OF FAT	MUFA	PUFA	SFA
Vegetable			
Canola (rapeseed)	66	24	5
Coconut	6	2	87
Corn	25	59	13
Olive	74	8	14
Palm	37	9	49
Peanut	46	32	17
Safflower	12	75	9
Soybean	23	58	14
Animal			
Beef	43	4	40
Butter	29	4	62
Chicken	39	22	28
Lamb	42	7	42
Pork	46	11	36
Salmon	35	29	19
Turkey	32	27	29

SFA, saturated fatty acids; MUFA, monounsaturated fatty acids; PUFA, polyunsaturated fatty acids.
Adapted from Agriculture Handbook, No. 8 Series, U.S. Department of Agriculture, Human Information Service
*These figures do not total 100%. Additional components include cholesterol and phytosterols.

CARBOHYDRATE AND FAT

With protein accounting for 10–20% of total calories, the remaining calories will be divided between carbohydrate and fat. The proportion derived from either depends on the medical outcome desired for each patient. Lipid abnormalities common in type II diabetes are influenced by both dietary carbohydrate and fat content, as well as weight, heredity, exercise, and glycemic control. Hypertriglyceridemia, the most common lipid abnormality in type II diabetes, is considered a significant risk factor for cardiovascular disease.

High carbohydrate intake (regardless of source) in susceptible people will increase postprandial and fasting triglyceride levels. This attribute has sparked concern about whether restricting dietary fat to <30% of calories, when 50–60% will then be carbohydrate in-take, is a judicious recommendation for patients with type II diabetes. Several studies suggest that a higher-fat diet (up to 40%) can improve serum lipids as well as or better than fat restriction, provided that the additional fat is predominately monounsaturated fatty acids (MUFA). Because major sources of MUFA are olive, canola, and peanut oils, increasing fat intake beyond substituting these oils in cooking may be difficult. In addition, olives, avocados, and nuts need to be incorporated into meals and snacks in receptive individuals.

Polyunsaturated fatty acids (PUFAs) are predominant in plant oils (corn, safflower, cottonseed, soy) and marine life. When substituted for saturated fat, PUFA lowers serum cholesterol, particularly LDL cholesterol. Fish oil contains PUFA in the form of ω-3 fatty acids. The ω-3 fatty acids have been found to specifically reduce serum triglycerides and decrease platelet aggregation. Although this is appealing to individuals with type II diabetes, clinical trials illustrate that fish-oil-capsule supplementation increases blood glucose levels. Consuming 8 oz fish/wk has been suggested to be both safe and potentially protective. All fish contains some fish oil, although salmon, albacore tuna, mackerel, and herring are the best sources.

Saturated fat in the diet should make up <10% of total calories. Saturated fat has been shown to be highly atherogenic and to have a greater impact on total and LDL cholesterol than does dietary cholesterol intake itself. Saturated fat is derived primarily from animal sources but varies between species (Table 3.4). Coconut and palm oil are also highly saturated and should be avoided. Limiting red meat intake to 3–4 oz/day, consuming skim milk, and substituting margarine for butter are acceptable ways to meet this 10% guideline. Controversy exists over whether stick margarines are a good substitute for butter, because the transfatty acids formed in the hydrogenation of vegetable oils to margarine may be as atherogenic as saturated fats. Soft, tub, and liquid margarines are a judicious choice until this question is answered.

Cholesterol intake should be limited to <300 mg/day. All animal products contain cholesterol, including meat, poultry, shellfish, eggs, and cheese. However, total and saturated fat are very low in poultry and fish; thus, they are the preferred choices for antiatherogenic diets.

It is well documented that large amounts of dietary fat contribute to the development and maintenance of obesity. Not only does fat contain more than twice as many calories as either carbohydrate or protein (9, 4, and 4 cal, respectively), but it is thought to be more easily converted to body fat. Because most individuals with type II diabetes are obese, it seems reasonable that restricting total dietary fat intake should be a nutrition goal. In addition, abnormal levels of LDL and total cholesterol are often associated with obesity and diabetes. Fat restriction to as low as 10–30% of calories can decrease both abnormalities. Weight loss also improves both hypercholesterolemia and hypertriglyceridemia. The resulting dilemma of the most appropriate level of fat intake for an obese individual with type II diabetes is best solved through metabolic evaluation. If a low-fat, low-calorie nutrition plan is not producing desired metabolic outcomes such as weight loss, decreased lipids, and good metabolic control, then fat intake could be increased by use of monounsaturated fat. The resulting decrease in carbohydrate intake may decrease both postprandial glycemia and hypertriglyceridemia. Periodic evaluations of therapy are essential to modifying the nutrition plan.

The Food Guide Pyramid serves as a model for recommending carbohydrate choices for individuals with type II diabetes. The emphasis on whole grains, starches, fruits, and vegetables supplies necessary fiber, vitamins, and minerals to the meal plan. Although fiber does not have a great effect on blunting blood glucose response, it has been shown to have hypocholesterolemic effects. In addition, fiber maintains normal gastrointestinal motility that becomes increasingly important with age. The Food Guide Pyramid and American Diabetes Association nutrition recommendations also allow for a modest amount of sugar in the daily diet when desired. Traditionally, starches and grains were thought to produce lower blood glucose responses than sugar-containing foods because of their more complex molecular structure. Clinical research, however, has shown that this is not true. Much of the blood glucose response is contingent on the speed of digestion. For example, liquids are absorbed rapidly and increase blood glucose quickly. Carbohydrate (wheat starch) found in bread may be more rapidly absorbed than wheat starch found in pasta and will produce a quicker blood glucose response. Factors such as the presence of fat, degree of ripeness, cooking method, and preparation may all affect the speed of digestion.

Including sugar in the meal plan may improve dietary adherence and quality of life in older type II diabetic adults who most likely have included these foods routinely throughout their life. Individuals should be taught how to appropriately substitute sugar-containing foods for other carbohydrates. SMBG can be used to evaluate the results and guide further modifications. Caution should be used recommending sugar-containing foods for obese individuals. Although deprivation is undesirable and can often lead to binging, limiting sweets to one small portion daily may trigger overconsumption in someone who may have little self-control. Individualizing the plan and close follow-up help to minimize this problem.

ALTERNATIVE SWEETENERS AND FAT SUBSTITUTES

Sorbitol, mannitol, and fructose are commonly used sweeteners that have a lower glycemic effect than either glucose or sucrose (table sugar). Because they contain the same amount of calories as glucose and sucrose (4 cal/g), they cannot be used ad libitum, particularly in the hypocaloric diet. The sugar alcohols sorbitol and mannitol may have only 2–3 cal/g, but are often found in products with large amounts of fat. They may cause bloating and diarrhea when more than 30 g/day are consumed (10–15 hard candies). Foods containing these sugars must be accounted for in the meal plan.

Noncaloric sweeteners such as aspartame, saccharin, and acesulfame K are 200 times sweeter than sugar. They are used in such small quantities that they contribute virtually no calories or nutrition to foods. Their use as tabletop sweeteners and in soft drinks is beneficial in diabetes because no calories or carbohydrates are contributed. However, they may be included in foods that usually contain other sources of carbohydrates and calories such as ice cream, cookies, and puddings. These foods need to be worked into the meal plan appropriately.

Fat substitutes currently on the market are derived primarily from carbohydrate or protein. This reduces their caloric value from 9 to 4 cal/g. However, the use of these foods in yogurt, ice cream, salad dressings, etc., increases the carbohydrate content of the products above their usual level. Individuals should be advised to consider the carbohydrate level when substituting and using such foods.

VITAMINS/MINERALS

There is no evidence for an increased need for vitamins or minerals in diabetes above the current RDA. However, antioxidants such as β-carotene, vitamin E, and vitamin C have been implicated as potentially valuable in reducing atherosclerotic lesions and cataracts—both of which are prevalent in type II diabetes. It is impossible through food intake to obtain the levels of vitamin E that studies show to be beneficial (100 IU/day). If the patient and physician feel supplementation is beneficial, vitamin E is considered safe at this level.

Sodium recommendations for people with diabetes are no more restrictive than for the general population. Some health authorities recommend no more than 3000 mg/day of sodium for the general population, whereas other authorities recommend no more than 2400 mg/day. For people with mild to moderate hypertension, $\leq$ 2400 mg/day of sodium is recommended. Severe sodium restriction seems to be less important than weight loss in controlling hypertension in obese patients with type II diabetes.

ALCOHOL

Strict abstinence from alcohol is not necessary for patients with diabetes mellitus. In most cases, moderate amounts of alcohol as recommended for the general population are allowed with diabetes. When alcohol is part of the meal plan, it is convenient to account for the calories by reducing the patient's fat intake. Before a patient may include alcohol in his/her eating plan, the potential problems associated with alcohol consumption should be considered; e.g., alcohol consumption by a person who is fasting (>5 h) or undernourished may lead to hypoglycemia. This can be a serious problem in patients taking insulin or an oral hypoglycemic agent who skip meals. A patient's ability to follow the prescribed management plan will be impaired if he/she is intoxicated.

Alcohol ingestion may be associated with significant elevations in fasting and postprandial plasma triglyceride levels. Because of the increased risk of cardiovascular disease in diabetes, alcohol consumption should probably be avoided if the patient has severe hypertriglyceridemia.

BIBLIOGRAPHY

American Diabetes Association consensus statement: Detection and management of lipid disorders in diabetes. *Diabetes Care* 16 (Suppl. 2):106–12, 1993

American Diabetes Association consensus statement: Role of cardiovascular risk factors in prevention and treatment of macrovascular disease in diabetes. *Diabetes Care* 12: 573–79, 1989

American Diabetes Association position statement: Nutrition recommendations and principles for people with diabetes mellitus. *Diabetes Care* 17:519–22, 1994

American Dietetic Association position statement: Use of nutritive and non-nutritive sweeteners. *J Am Diet Assoc* 93:816–21, 1993

Bantle JP, Swanson JE, Thomas W, Laine DC: Metabolic effects of dietary sucrose in type II diabetic subjects. *Diabetes Care* 16:1301, 1993

DCCT Research Group: Expanded role of the dietitian in the Diabetes Control and Complications Trial: implications for clinical practice. *J Am Diet Assoc* 93:758–64, 767, 1993

Franz MJ, Horton ES, Bantle JP, Beebe CA, Brunzell JD, Coulston AM, Henry RR, Hoogwerf BJ, Stacpoole PW: Nutrition principles for the management of diabetes and related complications. *Diabetes Care* 17: 490–518, 1994

Henry RR: Protein and diabetes mellitus. *Diabetes Care*. In press

Henry RR, Wallace P, Olefsky JM: Effects of weight loss on mechanisms of hyperglycemia in obese non-insulin-dependent diabetes mellitus. *Diabetes* 35:990–98, 1986

Nuttall FQ: Diet and the diabetic patient. *Diabetes Care* 6:197–207, 1983

Parillo M, Rivellese AA, Ciardullo AV, Capaldo B, Giacco A, Genovese S, Riccardi G: A high-monounsaturated fat/low carbohydrate diet improves peripheral insulin sensitivity in non-insulin dependent diabetic patients. *Metabolism* 41:1371–78, 1992

U.S. Department of Agriculture: *The Food Guide Pyramid.* Hyattsville, MD, Human Nutrition Information Service, 1992

Wing RR, Shoemaker M, Marcus MD, McDermott M, Gooding W: Variables associated with weight loss and improvements in glycemic control in type II diabetic patients in behavioral weight control programs. *Int J Obes* 14:495–503, 1990

Exercise

INTRODUCTION

Exercise in type II diabetes is an important management tool. To be effective, establishing and maintaining an exercise regimen requires individualization and monitoring. Specific precautions need to be taken in some individuals to ensure maximum benefits.

Both obesity and inactivity contribute to the development of glucose intolerance in the genetically predisposed individual. Current research suggests that regular exercise can delay or prevent type II diabetes in such high-risk populations. People with type II diabetes can experience several benefits from regular exercise.

POTENTIAL BENEFITS OF EXERCISE

Because type II diabetes occurs primarily in adults, many of the benefits relate to lifestyle changes and the related health outcomes. Regular exercise in type II diabetes can potentially

- reduce cardiovascular risk factors such as high blood levels of cholesterol or triglycerides, high blood pressure, and poor circulation;
- augment weight-reduction diets in promoting and maintaining weight loss;
- improve blood glucose control by enhancing insulin sensitivity;
- reduce dosage or need for insulin or oral hypoglycemic agents;
- enhance quality of life by improving muscle strength and joint flexibility; and
- improve psychological well-being and reduce stress.

Improved Insulin Sensitivity/ Glucose Tolerance

Insulin resistance is a hallmark of type II diabetes mellitus. Exercise enhances insulin sensitivity and increases skeletal muscle glucose uptake not only during but also after the activity. Enhanced insulin sensitivity dissipates within 48 h after exercise. Thus, repeated bouts of exercise at regular intervals are most beneficial to reduce the glucose intolerance associated with type II diabetes. This exercise-induced enhanced sensitivity to insulin occurs without changes in body weight. Unless contraindicated, exercise should be a component of the treatment regimen in all people with type II diabetes regardless of weight.

Exercise may decrease the necessary amount of insulin or oral hypoglycemic agent. Therefore, careful SMBG is required to minimize hypoglycemia and facilitate weight loss, if desired.

Exercise and Weight Reduction

Physical activity is recognized as an important part of weight-reduction programs. In fact, exercise has been identified consistently as the strongest predictor for long-term maintenance of lost weight. Exercise increases energy expenditure to create a greater calorie deficit than a hypocaloric diet alone. Exercise also increases lean body mass (muscle tissue), which helps to maintain the metabolic rate that otherwise declines with loss of body weight. Of particular importance is that aerobic exercise decreases abdominal (central) adiposity. Because central obesity increases cardiovascular risk, this can be a valuable benefit in patients with type II diabetes.

Cardiovascular Benefits

The value of physical training in ameliorating risk factors for cardiovascular disease has been amply demonstrated in nondiabetic individuals. Exercise is associated with a reduction in circulating levels of very-low-density lipoprotein and LDL cholesterol, triglycerides, and insulin. Exercise also is associated with increases in HDL cholesterol, which may provide protection against cardiovascular disease. Furthermore, exercise is associated with decreases in blood pressure and heart rate both at rest and during exercise, as well as increases in maximum oxygen uptake and total working capacity.

The beneficial effects of exercise on risk factors in patients with type II diabetes have not been studied extensively, but it is reasonable to assume that exercise may help to prevent or retard cardiovascular complications in this particularly susceptible group of individuals. Again, however, the cardiovascular and metabolic benefits of exercise are sustained only as the result of the sum of effects of individual bouts of exercise or as a result of long-term changes in body composition.

Psychological Benefits

Exercise training and fitness are often associated with decreased anxiety, improved mood and self-esteem, and an increased sense of well-being. Enhanced quality of life may be a secondary benefit to strength training (increased muscle mass, flexibility, range of motion), particularly in the aging population, in which type II diabetes predominates. Regular exercise is considered an important stress management technique as well. Regular exercise may improve glucose control in part by providing a coping mechanism for stress.

PRECAUTIONS AND CONSIDERATIONS

Exercise of any kind is safe for most people with type II diabetes. However, special precautions should be taken. Because many individuals with type II diabetes have led sedentary lives for years, they are frequently deconditioned. Individuals over age 35 yr not engaged in regular exercise should have a physical examination (including a stress test) before beginning to exercise.

The medical evaluation should include the following:
■ determination of glycemic control
■ cardiovascular examination (blood pressure, peripheral pulses, bruits, blood lipids, ECG at rest and during exercise if the patient is >35 yr old or has a history of cardiovascular disease);
■ determination of working capacity (graduated exercise test with measurement of pulse-rate response or oxygen consumption);
■ neurologic examination;
■ ophthalmoscopic examination; and
■ detailed ophthalmologic evaluation if proliferative retinopathy is present or suspected.

Most people with type II diabetes have had the disease an average of 7 yr before diagnosis, and newly diagnosed patients should be examined for diabetes complications such as hypertension, neuropathy, retinopathy, and nephropathy (Table 3.5). Silent ischemic heart disease can be present without chest pain. Therefore, it is prudent to consider whether autonomic neuropathy is present before setting exercise goals. Autonomic neuropathy and β-blockers may also interfere with maximal heart rate and exercise performance. This is in addition to the already observed 15–20% lower age-matched maximal heart rate found in people with type II diabetes. Lower target heart rates and less stressful exercise regimens are recommended in these individuals. Strenuous exercise is contraindicated for patients with poor metabolic control and for those with significant diabetic complications (particularly active proliferative retinopathy, significant cardiovascular disease, and neuropathy).

Foot sensitivity and adequacy of circulation should be evaluated, and those with evidence of problems with either should avoid forms of exercise that involve trauma to the feet. Proper foot wear is important when patients with type II diabetes engage in exercise.

Most patients with active proliferative retinopathy and or hypertension should avoid strenuous, high-intensity exercises associated with Valsalva-like maneuvers, e.g., weight lifting and certain types of isometrics. Rhythmic exercises involving the lower extremities, e.g., walking, jogging, swimming, and cycling, are generally preferred for patients with hypertension.

Prolonged exercise can potentiate the hypoglycemic effects of both oral agents and insulin. Hypoglycemia can occur during or as much as 12 h after the exer-

Table 3.5. Precautions for Patients With Medical Complications

■ Insensitive feet or peripheral vascular insufficiency: avoid running; choose walking, cycling, swimming; emphasize proper footwear.

■ Untreated or recently treated proliferative retinopathy: avoid exercises associated with increased intra-abdominal pressure, Valsalva-like maneuvers, or rapid head movements or eye trauma.

■ Hypertension: avoid heavy lifting and Valsalva-like maneuvers; choose exercises that primarily involve the lower-extremity rather than upper-extremity muscle groups.

cise session. SMBG in response to exercise is beneficial in guiding medication adjustments to prevent hypoglycemia. Insulin may need to be decreased on days during which exercise is performed (Table 3.6). This is particularly important if exercise is an adjunct to weight loss. It would be counterproductive to have to treat a hypoglycemic reaction with food or to consume extra food to prevent hypoglycemia in patients on a hypocaloric diet.

Special precautions should be taken when the patient requires or uses drugs that may make him/her more susceptible to exercise-inducted hypoglycemia. For example, alcohol and very high doses of salicylates should be avoided because they may themselves produce hypoglycemia. The β-adrenergic–blocking agents may prevent the rapid hepatic glyconeolytic responses that normally correct hypoglycemia. Certain other drugs, including bishydroxycoumarin, phenylbutazone, sulfonamides, and monoamine oxidase inhibitors, may potentiate the action of sulfonylurea agents.

Patients with type II diabetes controlled by diet alone can perform exercise in the same manner as people without diabetes. Supplementary food before, during, or after activity is unnecessary, because hypoglycemia is not a risk.

THE EXERCISE PRESCRIPTION

The key to a successful exercise program is individualization. The exercise program must be designed with the patient in mind and take into account the interests, initial physical condition, and motivation of the patient. A safe exercise prescription is based on a complete medical evaluation and requires that special instructions be given to the patient for managing the exercise program. The patient should start slowly, exercise at regular intervals at least 3–4 times weekly, and gradually increase the duration and intensity of the exercise. Timing the exercise session in type II diabetes may be used advantageously. It appears that exercise performed after 1600 h may reduce hepatic glucose output and decrease fasting glycemia. Exercise after eating may reduce postprandial hyperglycemia common in type II diabetes. Because exercise is so important, it should be encouraged regardless of when it is performed.

Activity

The type of exercise a patient chooses to perform should be tailored to his/her physical capacity and interests. Most patients can, at minimum, undertake a walking program safely. Aerobic activities, e.g., biking, swimming, jogging, and dancing, should be encouraged as well. Biking and swimming are particularly valuable in patients with neuropathy, where foot placement and steady gait may be compromised.

A complete exercise program also includes muscle-strengthening exercises such as lifting light weights. Armchair exercises can be performed by individuals who are confined to a chair or who may have limited mobility. Flexibility-type stretches are useful during warm-up and cool-down periods. These not only prepare muscles for an aerobic workout but also promote improved range of motion, which is especially valuable in elderly people.

Intensity

There are several ways to monitor exercise intensity. One recommendation is to sustain a heart rate at ~60–80% of the maximal heart rate. Working out at even 50% may be beneficial. Previously sedentary patients should never be given a high-end heart rate goal unless an exercise stress test is performed. However, a low-end heart rate goal, i.e., stay <110 beats/min, can be given before stress testing. Another alternative is to use a rating of perceived exertion: patients can be guided to work hard—generally a brisk pace where a light sweat may be present and they perceive they are working. At this pace, they should have enough breath to carry on a conversation. In general, patients should not focus primarily on the intensity of activity, because any activity is preferred to a sedentary lifestyle.

Duration

The vigorous or aerobic portion of an exercise session should last a minimum of 20 min, with a goal of 30–40 min. This should be preceded by a 5- to 10 min warm-up period and followed by a 5- to 10-min cool-down period. These warm-up and cool-down periods may include some weight lifting and flexibility exercise. Most patients will need to work up to this gradually with as little as a 5-min aerobic period that increases incrementally by 1–2 min every 1–2 wk.

Frequency

The benefits of exercise in type II diabetes are achieved by sustained repeated bouts of activity ≤48 h apart. Thus, for fitness, exercise should be performed at least 3 times/wk or every other day. Weight reduction is enhanced by exercise sessions performed nearly 5–6 times per wk.

BIBLIOGRAPHY

American Diabetes Association position statement: Diabetes mellitus and exercise. *Diabetes Care* 16 (Suppl. 2):37, 1993

American Diabetes Association technical review: Exercise and NIDDM. *Diabetes Care* 16 (Suppl. 2):54–58, 1993

Table 3.6. Guidelines for Safe Exercise

- Carry an identification card and wear a bracelet, necklace, or tag at all times that identifies them as having diabetes
- If the patient uses insulin:
  - Avoid exercise during peak insulin action
  - Administer insulin away from working limbs
  - If patient takes single daily dose of intermediate-acting insulin, decrease dose by as much as 30–35% or shift to a schedule of ≥2 doses/day, with or without addition of short-acting insulin, on days when exercise is planned
  - If patient uses combination of short- and intermediate-acting insulin, decrease or omit short-acting insulin dose and decrease dose of intermediate-acting insulin by up to one third on days when exercise is planned; this may produce hyperglycemia later in the day that requires a second injection of short-acting insulin
  - If patient uses only short-acting insulin, reduce the preexercise dose; reduce the postexercise dose based on self-monitoring of blood glucose; total dose may need to be reduced by as much as 30–50% on days when exercise is planned
- Be alert for signs of hypoglycemia during and for several hours after exercise
- Have immediate access to a source of readily absorbable carbohydrate (such as glucose tablets) to treat hypoglycemia
- If preexercise fasting blood glucose is >300 mg/dl (16.7 mM), delay exercising until glucose is controlled
- Take sufficient fluids before, after, and if necessary, during exercise to prevent dehydration.

Campaigne BN, Lampman RM: *Exercise in the Clinical Management of Diabetes.* Champaign, IL, Human Kinetics, 1994

Fitness Book for People With Diabetes. Hornsby GH, Ed. Alexandria, VA, Am. Diabetes Assoc., 1994

Gordon NF: *Diabetes: Your Complete Exercise Guide.* Champaign, IL, Human Kinetics, 1993

Graham C, Lasko-McCarthey P: Exercise options for persons with diabetic complications. *Diabetes Educator* 16:212–20, 1990

Maynard T: Exercise. Pt. I. Physiological response to exercise in diabetes mellitus. *Diabetes Educator* 17:196–206, 1991

Maynard T: Exercise. Pt II. Translating the exercise prescription. *Diabetes Educator* 17:384–95, 1991

Pharmacologic Intervention

INTRODUCTION

Pharmacologic intervention should only be considered when the patient with type II diabetes cannot achieve normal or near-normal plasma glucose levels with nutrition therapy and regular exercise. The two options for this stage of therapy are oral hypoglycemic agents and insulin. The question is, Which pharmacologic alternative is best for the patient? The physician can determine the answer to this question, in part, by considering the following:

- the severity of the patient's disease (i.e., degree of hyperglycemia, presence/absence of symptoms);
- the condition of the patient otherwise (presence/absence of concurrent diseases and conditions);
- the preferences of the patient who has been well informed about the use, expected therapeutic effects, and possible side effects of oral agents and insulin;
- the patient's ability for self-care management;
- the motivation of the patient; and
- the age and weight of the patient.

TREATMENT WITH ORAL HYPOGLYCEMIC AGENTS

Oral hypoglycemic agents (sulfonylureas) are often therapeutically effective in patients with type II diabetes who have not met the goals of therapy after institution of dietary modification and exercise. The mechanism of action of sulfonylurea agents is complex. Sulfonylureas are only effective when there is endogenous insulin secretion. Acutely, they augment β-cell insulin secretion. After several months of therapy, however, insulin levels return to pretreatment values, whereas glucose levels remain improved. Sulfonylurea compounds may reduce the accelerated rates of hepatic glucose production in type II diabetes and may partially reverse defects in insulin action. The relative importance of each of these actions in ameliorating hyperglycemia is unclear, but it is likely that pancreatic effects are required.

The use of an oral hypoglycemic agent should be considered seriously only if it is clear that there are no contraindications to its use. For example, oral hypoglycemic agents require the presence of endogenous insulin and therefore are ineffective and contraindicated for patients with type I diabetes mellitus. In addition, oral agents should not be used during pregnancy and lactation because the effects of oral agents on the fetus and/or newborn are unknown. Similarly, oral hypoglycemic agents are generally not recommended for seriously ill patients or patients with kidney and liver disease. Finally, oral hypoglycemic agents are contraindicated in patients who are known to be allergic to sulfa drugs.

A new oral hypoglycemic agent, metformin, will likely become available in the United States. This biguanide has been used extensively in Europe and Canada for >20 yr. It has a different structure and mode of action than the sulfonylurea drugs.

Clinical Use of Oral Hypoglycemic Agents

To use these agents most appropriately, it is useful to consider them in terms of effectiveness, pharmacokinetics, and metabolism, as well as possible complications, factors that influence choice of agents, guidelines for prescription, and possible reasons for drug failure (Table 3.7).

Tolbutamide (Orinase). Tolbutamide is a short-acting sulfonylurea drug that is usually taken 2 or 3 times per day. This drug is metabolized by the liver to totally inactive products that are excreted in the urine. Therefore, this drug may be useful in some patients with mild renal impairment. Because of its short half-life and the fact that it therefore needs to be taken 2–3 times a day, compliance may be a problem.

Chlorpropamide (Diabinese). Chlorpropamide is partially metabolized by the liver to metabolites that retain hypoglycemic activity, and these metabolites plus intact drug are excreted in the urine. Chlorpropamide has the longest duration of action (~60 h) and is only given once per day. This compound can cause significant hyponatremia. In addition, a mild Antabuse-like reaction (alcohol flushing) can occur with this agent.

Tolazamide (Tolinase). Tolazamide is an intermediate-duration sulfonylurea compound that is metabolized by the liver. The by-products of metabolism have relatively little hypoglycemic activity and are excreted in the urine. Tolazamide is usually taken once or twice a day.

Glipizide (Glucotrol and Glucotrol XL). This sulfonylurea is taken once or twice a day and has a duration of action of 12–24 h. It is metabolized by the liver to inactive products that are excreted in the urine. A long-acting sustained-release preparation of glipizide is also available (XL).

Glyburide (Diabeta, Micronase, and Glynase PresTab). This sulfonylurea has a duration of action of 16–24 h. It can be given once or twice a day. It is metabolized by the liver to several weakly active and inactive derivatives that are excreted in the urine and the bile. A micronized (small particle size) tablet is available that facilitates rapid absorption of the drug (Glynase PresTab).

Metformin (Glucophage). This guanidine derivative decreases blood glucose levels in type II diabetic patients primarily by an increase in glucose utilization; it does not stimulate insulin secretion. Metformin is not associated with hypoglycemic reactions or weight gain and is usually used alone or combined with sulfonylureas to control hyperglycemia in patients who have primary or secondary failure with sulfonylereas alone. Associated with metformin treatment in type II diabetic patients are decreases in triglyceride and low-density lipoprotein cholesterol levels. The major side effects of metformin, which occur in 10–30% of patients, are gastrointestinal and include anorexia, nausea, abdominal discomfort, and diarrhea. These side effects lessen with chronic therapy. Lactic acidosis is a rare complication with metformin therapy; however, metformin should not be given to patients with kidney or liver desease, alcohol abuse, or cardiorespiratory insufficiency. It is contraindicated during pregnancy.

Complications of Sulfonylurea Therapy

Major concerns about the cardiovascular risk of oral hypoglycemic agents, which were raised in 1970 when the University Group Diabetes Program (UGDP) study was published, have diminished because there is no agreement on interpretation of data from that study. Problems with study design make a valid interpretation of the UGDP data difficult. Moreover, similar studies could not confirm these findings.

The major benefit of the UGDP study was to focus attention on treatment of type II diabetes in general and on the appropriate use of oral hypoglycemic agents in particular. As a result of the study, most clinicians agree that the cornerstone of therapy for type II diabetes is dietary modification plus regular exercise and that the use of any pharmacologic agent is an adjunct to rather than a substitute for dietary modification and exercise.

Severe hypoglycemia is the major complication of sulfonylurea therapy and has been a particular problem with chlorpropamide because of its long duration of action. Elderly patients are more susceptible to hypoglycemia, particularly when they have a tendency to skip meals or when renal function is impaired. Severe hypoglycemia may also occur in individuals who consume alcohol and skip meals.

Side effects are uncommon, but the predominant ones are gastrointestinal effects (e.g., nausea and vomiting) and skin reactions (e.g., rashes, purpura, and pruritus). Other side effects of sulfonylurea agents include hematologic reactions (leukopenia, thrombocytopenia, hemolytic anemia) and cholestasis (with and without jaundice). Cholestatic jaundice has been identified more often with

Table 3.7. Characteristics of Oral Hypoglycemic Agents

GENERIC NAME	BRAND NAME	DAILY DOSAGE RANGE (mg)	DURATION OF ACTION (h)	COMMENTS
Tolbutamide	Orinase	500–3000	6–12	Metabolized by liver to an inactive product; excreted by kidneys; given 2–3 times per day
Chlorpropamide	Diabinese	100–500	60	Metabolized by liver (~70%) to less active metabolites and excreted intact (~30%) by kidneys; can potentiate antidiuretic hormone action; given once per day
Tolazamide	Tolinase	100–1000	12–24	Metabolized by liver to both active and inactive products; excreted by kidneys; given 1–2 times per day
Glipizide	Glucotrol	2.5–40	12–24	Metabolized by liver to inert products; excreted by kidneys; given 1–2 times per day
	Glucotrol XL	5–20	24	A preparation that allows controlled release, which produces sustained plasma levels
Glyburide	Diabeta, Micronase	1.25–20	16–24	Metabolized by liver to mostly inert products; excreted in bile and by kidneys; given 1–2 times per day
	Glynase PresTab	0.75–12	12–24	The small particle size of this glyburide preparation facilitates rapid absorption
Metformin	Glucophage	1500–2500	*	Not metabolized; excreted by kidneys; may be used alone or in combination therapy.

*Plasma elimination half-life is ~5.5 h.

the use of chlorpropamide than with any other oral agent. Chlorpropamide also facilitates antidiuretic hormone secretion and action. Chlorpropamide-induced hyponatremia is particularly common in elderly patients, especially when given in combination with thiazide diuretics. For these reasons, chlorpropamide is generally not appropriate as a first-line therapy.

There are many drugs that can potentiate or interfere with the hypoglycemic action of sulfonylurea drugs. Sulfonylurea drugs bind to serum proteins via ionic (tolbutamide, chlorpropamide, tolazamide) and nonionic (glipizide and glyburide) mechanisms. Other drugs may alter the affects of sulfonylureas. The clinical significance of these effects on glycemic control are unknown. Table 3.8 lists some of the most important of these drugs; their administration with sulfonylureas must be carefully monitored.

Choice of Agent

Four criteria should be considered when choosing the appropriate sulfonylurea:
- efficacy;
- complications, i.e., duration of action;
- ease of compliance, i.e., number of doses per day, availability; and
- price.

When all factors are considered, glyburide, glipizide, and metformin are the most reasonable choices for most patients.

Drug Administration

After the most appropriate agent is selected for a particular patient, the lowest recommended dose should be prescribed. The dose should be increased every 1–2 wk until satisfactory glycemic control or the maximum dose is reached. Too often, clinicians stop short once symptoms are relieved rather than raising doses in an attempt to reach treatment goals. If the maximum dose of the initially selected agent does not provide adequate glycemic control, then the patient is a candidate for insulin therapy. No benefit is achieved by using two sulfonylurea drugs simultaneously.

Drug Failures

Most patients with type II diabetes demonstrate an initial satisfactory response to sulfonylurea therapy. When a patient does not respond initially, this is called primary failure. When initial glycemic control is achieved with an oral agent and then lost, the patient is considered a secondary drug failure. Secondary drug failure occurs in 5–10% of patients per year, depending on the characteristics of the population studied. In some cases, secondary failure occurs because the patient does not follow the prescribed diet, and correction of dietary indiscretion can restore the desired glycemic effect of the drug. In other

Table 3.8. Drugs That Alter Sulfonylurea Action

DRUGS THAT ENHANCE HYPOGLYCEMIC ACTIVITY

Affect sulfonylurea pharmacokinetics
- Displacement from albumin binding site
- Clofibrate
- Halofenate
- Phenylbutazone, oxyphenylbutazone, and sulfinpyrazone
- Salicylates
- Some sulfonamides
- Prolong half-life by interfering with metabolism
  - Bihydroxycoumarin
  - Chloramphenicol
  - Monoamine oxidase inhibitors
  - Pyrazolone derivatives (e.g., phenylbutazone)
- Decrease urinary excretion
  - Allopurinol
  - Probenecid
  - Pyrazolone derivatives (e.g., phenylbutazone)
  - Some sulfonamides

Have their own intrinsic hypoglycemic activity
- Alcohol
- Guanethidine
- Monoamine oxidase inhibitors
- Salicylates

DRUGS THAT ANTAGONIZE SULFONYLUREA ACTION AND CAUSE HYPERGLYCEMIA

Shorten sulfonylurea half-life by increasing metabolism
- Chronic alcohol use
- Rifampin

Have own intrinsic hyperglycemic activity
- Acetazolamide
- β-Blockers
- Diazoxide
- Diuretics (e.g., thiazides, furosemide)
- Epinephrine
- Glucagon
- Glucocorticoids
- Indomethacin
- Isoniazid
- Nicotinic acid
- Phenytoin
- Progestins
- L-Thyroxine

cases of secondary failure, progression of disease should be considered, as should the occurrence of an underlying stressful disease or condition, e.g., infection, pregnancy, or cardiovascular event. In these situations, the patient should be switched to insulin. After recovery from an intercurrent disease or condition, reinstitution of oral hypoglycemic therapy may be successful.

INSULIN THERAPY

Insulin is capable of restoring glycemia to near normal in most patients with type II diabetes. Although this therapy may result in elevated insulin levels, the relationship, if any, between hyperinsulinemia and long-term diabetes complications is unknown. In contrast, there is clear evidence that hyperglycemia exacerbates diabetes complications. Therefore, the focus should be on glucose control rather than on the theoretical deleterious effects of hyperinsulinemia.

Some physicians prefer insulin to oral hypoglycemic agents as the primary pharmacologic intervention (i.e., after diet and exercise have failed to normalize blood glucose). Insulin may be particularly appropriate as primary therapy in patients with rapid uncontrolled weight loss, unexplained by diet, who have severe hyperglycemia accompanied by ketonemia and/or ketonuria. Such patients may be severely insulin deficient and may, in fact, have type I diabetes. Other indications for the use of insulin include:
- hyperglycemia despite maximal doses of sulfonylureas;
- periods of acute injury, stress, infection, or surgery (in such circumstances, insulin requirements are increased, and dietary management with or without a concomitant oral hypoglycemic agent is generally inadequate);
- pregnancy;
- renal disease; and
- allergy or serious reaction to sulfa drugs.

Insulin therapy should be used with particular care in poorly compliant patients who are unwilling or unable to perform SMBG or in patients in whom hypoglycemia is a serious risk, e.g., patients with cerebrovascular disease or unstable angina. Note that any metabolic state or drug that increases requirements for insulin or interferes with insulin secretion may temporarily convert the patient with type II diabetes into an insulin-requiring patient. (Management of patients with insulin during pregnancy and surgery is discussed on pages 50–51.)

Insulin lowers the blood glucose level by increasing glucose uptake and metabolism by insulin-sensitive peripheral tissues (e.g., muscle and adipose tissue) and by suppressing hepatic glucose production. As with sulfonylureas, the improved glycemic control achieved with insulin therapy generally increases insulin action.

Because patients with type II diabetes are resistant to insulin action, they may require large doses of insulin to normalize their blood glucose. This may be particularly true for severely obese type II diabetic patients. Insulin is usually needed more than once a day. In some patients, a mixture of short- and intermediate-acting insulins may be required to achieve control.

Clinical Use of Insulin

Several important points about insulin therapy should be noted:
- Insulin treatment can be used to achieve near-normal blood glucose levels in patients with type II diabetes mellitus.
- Newly diagnosed patients with mild to moderately severe fasting hyperglycemia can be controlled with modest doses of insulin given once or several times a day.
- With time, insulin requirements may be expected to increase in patients with type II diabetes.
- When large doses of insulin are required or when there is a prominent glucose increase during the night, it is best to split the dose into ≥ 2 injections and to use a combination of short-acting insulin plus intermediate- or long-acting insulin.

Table 3.9. Time Course of Action of Insulin Preparations

INSULIN PREPARATION	ONSET OF ACTION	PEAK ACTION	DURATION OF ACTION
Short acting (regular)	30 min	2–5 h	5–8 h
Intermediate acting (NPH or lente)	1–3 h	6–12 h	16–24 h
Long acting (ultralente)	4–6 h	8–20 h	24–28 h
Mixtures (70/30, 50/50)	30 min	7–12 h	16–24 h

This table summarizes the typical time course of action of various insulin preparations. These values are highly variable among individuals. Even in a given patient, these values vary depending on the site and depth of injection, skin temperature, and exercise.

■ In some patients, regimens often recommended for type I diabetes, e.g., multiple injections, may be necessary to achieve target goals.

Types of Insulin

A wide variety of purified insulins are available. Beef insulin is considerably more antigenic than pork or human insulin. However, since the introduction of more purified insulin preparations, complications including delayed hyper-

Figure 3.1. Regulation of Glycemia by 2 Doses of Combined Short- and Intermediate-Acting Insulin

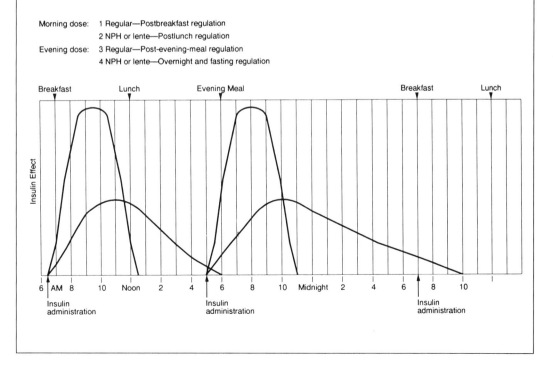

Morning dose: 1 Regular—Postbreakfast regulation
               2 NPH or lente—Postlunch regulation
Evening dose: 3 Regular—Post-evening-meal regulation
               4 NPH or lente—Overnight and fasting regulation

sensitivity, antibody-mediated insulin resistance, and lipoatrophy have become rare.

The selection of a specific insulin preparation is dictated by patient needs. Human insulin is the least antigenic and therefore may be preferred for patients with insulin allergy, severe insulin resistance due to insulin antibodies, or lipoatrophy. Patients who are candidates for intermittent insulin therapy (e.g., those who require insulin because of onset of diabetes during pregnancy or for acute problems such as infection, myocardial infarction, and emergency surgery) should be treated with human insulin to minimize the likelihood of insulin allergy or the ultimate development of insulin resistance. This theoretical advantage must be balanced against the generally shorter duration of action of human insulin, which may necessitate multiple daily injections.

Duration of Action

The selection of an appropriate insulin preparation also depends on the desired course of action. Table 3.9 summarizes the typical time course of action of various insulin preparations. However, these values are highly variable among individuals. Even in a given patient, these values vary depending on the site and depth of injection, skin temperature, and exercise. Some patients with mild to moderate fasting hyperglycemia may adequately control their condition with one injection of intermediate-acting insulin before breakfast or at bedtime. However, many patients need a second injection. This need is determined with SMBG and glycated hemoglobin.

Furthermore, SMBG records will help identify those patients who need the addition of short-acting insulin with either intermediate-acting or long-acting insulin (Figure 3.1).

Some individuals may have difficulty mixing insulins. For these patients, premixed insulins should be considered.

Table 3.10. Insulin Regimen and Timing of Self-Monitoring of Blood Glucose (SMBG)

INSULIN	TIME INJECTED	PERIOD OF ACTIVITY	SMBG REFLECTING INSULIN ACTION
Short acting	Before a meal	Between that meal and either the subsequent one or the bedtime snack (if insulin is taken before dinner)	Both after meal before which insulin is injected and before next meal or bedtime snack (if insulin is taken before dinner)
Intermediate acting	Before breakfast	Between lunch and dinner	Before dinner
Intermediate acting	Before dinner or bedtime	Overnight	Before breakfast
Long acting	Before breakfast *or* before dinner *or* half dose at each time	Mostly overnight because short acting insulin overrides its effect during the day	Before breakfast

Because the absorption of short-acting insulin is delayed when mixed with a lente preparation (due to the high zinc content of the latter), NPH insulin is the intermediate-acting insulin of choice.
Adapted from Davidson MB: How to get the most out of insulin therapy. *Clinical Diabetes* 8:65–73, 1990

Table 3.11. Sample Insulin Regimens for Achieving Glycemic Control

REGIMEN	BEFORE BREAKFAST	BEFORE LUNCH	BEFORE DINNER	BEFORE BEDTIME
1	Intermediate acting/ short acting*		Intermediate acting/ short acting	
2	Intermediate acting/ short acting		Short acting	Intermediate acting
3	Short acting	Short acting	Intermediate or long acting	
4	Short acting	Short acting	Short acting	Intermediate acting
5	Long acting†/short acting (separate injections)	Short-acting	Short acting	
6	Intermediate acting/ short acting*			

*Short-acting insulin should be injected 30 min before designated meal.
†May also be given either entirely at bedtime or before dinner or half the dose before breakfast and half before dinner.

However, care must be taken in adjusting the dose of premixed insulin.

Multidose Insulin Program

Doses of insulin are best adjusted according to SMBG values measured in the patient's usual environment. However, as in the DCCT, hospitalization for 2–3 days in a specialized metabolic setting may be used to initiate intensive treatment programs. The period during which glucose concentrations are controlled by various components of the insulin regimen and the timing of the tests reflecting that activity are shown in Table 3.10. Six different insulin regimens are shown in Table 3.11. In the first five, each component of the insulin regimen is reflected by the results of a different test. In the sixth, both the predinner and fasting glucose values reflect the activity of the morning intermediate-acting insulin. The glucose concentration before dinner usually decreases faster than the next day's fasting glucose level. As the dose of the morning intermediate-acting insulin is increased further to control the fasting value, unacceptable hypoglycemia often occurs in the late afternoon. If this should happen, a small dose of intermediate-acting insulin can be added in the evening (maintaining the dose of morning intermediate-acting insulin that led to acceptable predinner glucose values) and increased until the prebreakfast glucose level is appropriate.

The regimen with injections of short-acting insulin before each meal gives patients more flexibility with their eating and exercise patterns than the mixed-split regimen or the one with morning intermediate-acting insulin only.

Insulin doses vary widely among patients, even those of similar weight. A safe way to begin insulin is to start with an arbitrary dose and increase it gradually until the desired level of control is achieved. For lean patients (<125% desirable body wt), this might be 10 U intermediate-acting insulin in the morning and 5 U intermediate-acting insulin in the evening. In obese patients (>125% desirable body wt), the amounts would be higher (e.g., 20 and 10 U, respectively). The doses could be increased in 2- to 6-U increments depending on body weight and glucose levels at the appropriate times. It is better to adjust doses of short-acting insulin in the mixed-split regimen only after the prebreakfast and predinner glucose levels have decreased to more moderate values (e.g., <150 mg/dl [<8.3 mM]). For example, it would take much more short-acting insulin to lower a fasting glucose concentration of 240 mg/dl (13.3 mM) to an acceptable prelunch value in a patient just starting insulin than after the fasting value had been decreased to 120 mg/dl (6.7 mM). Short-acting insulin could be withheld or a small amount (2–4 U) given and held constant until that time.

The evening intermediate-acting insulin may be given before dinner. As the dose is increased to achieve a lower fasting glucose concentration, some patients will experience overnight hypoglycemia. If this should occur, moving the intermediate-acting insulin to bedtime usually corrects the problem, because the peak activity then occurs closer to breakfast.

If a regimen with injections of short-acting insulin before each meal is utilized, the initial dose might be 4 U for lean patients and 8 U for obese patients. The initial evening intermediate-acting insulin dose or total amount of long-acting insulin (whether given once per day or split in half) might be 10 U for lean patients and 16 U for obese patients. Gradual adjustments are made depending on the results of SMBG at the appropriate times (Table 3.10).

Dosage Requirements

The total dose of insulin needed by a patient with type II diabetes may be as little as 5–10 U/day or as much as several hundred units per day. Because insulin resistance is a significant component of both type II diabetes and obesity, it is evident that some obese patients with type II diabetes may require large quantities of insulin (>100 U/day) to control hyperglycemia appropriately. When smaller doses of insulin suffice (<30 U/day), a single injection of intermediate-acting insulin in the morning, or in some cases at bedtime, may be adequate. Alternately, two or more injections may be used when larger doses are required. (Table 3.11). Injection regimens should be tailored to the individual according to SMBG.

Complications of Insulin Therapy

The major complication of insulin therapy in patients with type II diabetes is the same as that in patients with type I diabetes, i.e., hypoglycemia. This complication may be managed by making changes in the dose or type of insulin used. The consequences of hypoglycemia may be greater in elderly patients. Lipodystrophies, antibody formation including insulin resistance, and allergy also occur but are uncommon with newer insulin preparations.

When insulin therapy is instituted as a multiple-dose regimen to effect tight control, greater attention should be paid to decreasing caloric intake.

COMBINATION THERAPY: INSULIN PLUS ORAL AGENT

Sulfonylurea drugs act by increasing insulin secretion and improving insulin action. Because of the latter, there may be some indication for combining insulin and sulfonylurea therapy in the same patient. However, there is limited evidence that combination therapy is more effective than multidose insulin regimens that have been fully optimized. Indeed, several retrospective analyses of the data have concluded that insulin-sulfonylurea therapy produces a level of glycemic control similar to insulin therapy alone, although less insulin is required. This is a theoretical but unproven advantage.

Studies evaluating the addition of sulfonylurea agents to the regimens of patients with type II diabetes who are inadequately controlled on insulin have shown only a minimal improvement in glycemic control (~1% decrease in glycated hemoglobin levels). These patients simply require more insulin. However, in patients failing maximal doses of sulfonylurea agents, addition of bedtime intermediate-acting insulin can be effective. With this approach of bedtime insulin/daytime sulfonylureas (BIDS), the evening intermediate-acting insulin controls the fasting glucose level, and the oral agent is used to control glucose levels during the day. Although some patients are reluctant to start insulin, many can be convinced to start BIDS because only one injection and one SMBG before breakfast are required. If the glycated hemoglobin reflects continued inadequate control, discontinuation of sulfonylurea agents and use of a mixed-split or other regimen should be used.

ADVERSE DRUG REACTIONS

There are several drugs in common use today that adversely affect diabetic patients because they may cause hyper- or hypoglycemia. These drugs should be prescribed with caution (Table 3.8).

BIBLIOGRAPHY

American Diabetes Association position statement: Insulin administration. *Diabetes Care* 16 (Suppl. 2):31–34, 1993

Furth FG, Bell PM, Rizza RA: Effects of tolazamide and exogenous insulin on insulin action in patients with noninsulin-dependent diabetes mellitus. *N Engl J Med* 314:1280–86, 1986

Galloway JA, de Shazo RD: Complications of insulin treatment. In *Diabetes Mellitus: Theory and Practice*. 4th ed. Rifkin H, Porte D, Eds. New York, Elsevier, 1990, p. 497–513

Genuth S: Insulin use in NIDDM. *Diabetes Care* 13:1240–64, 1990

Groop L, Groop P, Stenmar S, Saloranter C, Totterman K, Fyrquist F, Melander A: Comparison of pharmacokinetics, metabolic effects and mechanism of action of glyburide and glipizide during long-term treatment. *Diabetes Care* 10: 671– 78, 1987

Groop LC: Sulfonylureas in NIDDM. *Diabetes Care* 15:731–54, 1992

Lebovitz HE: Metformin. In Therapy for Diabetes Mellitus and Related Disorders. 2nd ed. Lebovitz HE, Ed. Alexandria, VA, Am. Diabetes Assoc., 1994, p. 124–27

Lebovitz HE: Oral hypoglycemic agents. In *Diabetes Mellitus: Theory and Practice*. 4th ed. Rifkin H, Porte D, Eds. New York, Elsevier, 1990, p. 554–74

Melander A: Clinical pharmacology of sulfonylureas. *Metabolism* 36 (Suppl. 1):12–16, 1987

Multicenter Study: UK prospective diabetes study. II. Reduction in HbA_{1c} with basal insulin supplement, sulfonylurea, or biguanide therapy in maturity-onset diabetes. *Diabetes* 34:793–98, 1985

Multicenter Study: UK prospective study of therapies of maturity-onset diabetes. I. Effect of diet, sulphonylurea, insulin or biguanide therapy on fasting plasma glucose and body weight over one year. *Diabetologia* 24:404–11, 1983

Pugh JA, Wager ML, Sawyer J, Ramirez G, Tinley M, Friedberg SJ: Is combination sulfonylurea and insulin therapy useful in NIDDM patients? A metaanalysis. *Diabetes Care* 15:953–59, 1992

Riddle MD: Evening insulin strategy. *Diabetes Care* 13:676–86, 1990

Scarlett JA, Gray RS, Griffin J, Olefsky JM, Kolterman OG: Insulin treatment reserves the insulin resistance of type II diabetes mellitus. *Diabetes Care* 5:353–63, 1982

Skyler JS: Insulin pharmacology. *Med Clin North Am* 72:1337–54, 1988

Stolar MW: Atherosclerosis in diabetes: the role of hyperinsulinemia. *Metabolism* 37 (Suppl. 1):1–9, 1988

University Group Diabetes Program: Effects of hypoglycemic agents on vascular complications in patients with adult-onset diabetes. VIII. Evaluation of insulin therapy: final report. *Diabetes* 31 (Suppl. 5):1–26, 1982

Yki-Jarvinen H, Kauppilia M, Kujansuu E, Lahti J, Marjanen T, Niskanen L, Rajala S, Rgyly L, Salo S, Seppala P, et al.: Comparison of insulin regimens in patients with non-insulin-dependent diabetes mellitus. *N Engl J Med* 327:1426–33, 1992

Special Therapeutic Problems

INTRODUCTION

Pregnancy and surgery in patients with diabetes are complicating situations that require extraordinary care to protect the patient against additional problems.

PREGNANCY

Pregnancy can cause clinical difficulties for both the patient and her unborn baby. The infant of a diabetic mother has an increased risk of death, prematurity, and morbidity (congenital defects, macrosomia, hypocalcemia, hyperbilirubinemia, and respiratory distress syndrome). The diabetic mother faces an increased risk of acceleration of microvascular complications involving the kidneys and eyes, particularly if hypertension is present.

In a patient with diabetes, pregnancy should be planned, so that conception occurs when the patient has normal fasting, preprandial, and postprandial plasma glucose levels. After conception, treatment should not only continue to achieve glycemic goals but also meet the nutritional requirements of the fetus. The patient who is treated with sulfonylureas should be switched to insulin therapy before conception. If the patient is being treated with a sulfonylurea agent and she becomes pregnant, she should be switched to insulin.

The physician should inform the patient of the risks to her and the baby. Because the risks of pregnancy in association with diabetes mellitus are great and involve both mother and fetus/newborn and the treatment program (multiple injections of insulin or use of the insulin pump and euglycemic regulation) is complex, the care of a pregnant diabetic woman should involve appropriate specialists. Consultation with a physician skilled in the care of pregnant diabetic women should be sought before conception or as soon as pregnancy is diagnosed to effect normalization of blood glucose levels.

Goals for glycemic control in diabetic women during pregnancy are:
- fasting, 60–90 mg/dl (3.3–5.0 mM),
- premeal, 60–105 mg/dl (3.3–5.8 mM),
- 1-h postprandial, 110–130 mg/dl (6.1–7.3 mM),
- 2-h postprandial, 90–120 mg/dl (5.0–6.7 mM), and
- 0200–0600, 60–120 mg/dl (3.3–6.7 mM).

The care of a pregnant diabetic woman requires a skilled health-care team. The physician who assumes responsibility for such a patient must be completely familiar with proper management of the patient and her fetus/newborn during pregnancy, just before and during delivery, and immediately after delivery. The same vigorous attention to glycemic regulation and proper management of the patient and her fetus/newborn must be given to the individual who develops gestational diabetes during the 2nd or 3rd trimester.

SURGERY

It is now possible for a patient with diabetes mellitus to undergo surgical operations with little more than normal risk, unless the operation is done under emergency conditions that do not allow complete evaluation and preparation of the patient. Proper surgical management of the diabetic candidate should be of concern to the physician in charge of a patient with type II diabetes mellitus. Conditions requiring surgery often develop in older people in general and in diabetic patients in particular (e.g., occlusive vascular disease, gallbladder disease, or cataract).

Unless the surgical condition is an emergency, the patient should be allowed sufficient time to achieve acceptable control of hyperglycemia before surgery. If possible, the patient should have a complete evaluation of metabolic state and thorough assessment of diabetic complications, including renal and cardiovascular disease, before surgery.

The objectives of management before, during, and after surgery are to prevent hypoglycemia, which can lead to coma, and to prevent excessive hyperglycemia and ketoacidosis, which can complicate postoperative care by causing dehydration, excessive protein loss, and electrolyte imbalance. To accomplish these ends, the anesthetic technique (regional or general) and the anesthetic agent should disrupt metabolic control as little as possible. Special attention should be given to maintaining proper fluid and electrolyte balance and blood glucose levels. Diabetic patients that have been treated with diet or oral agents may need insulin therapy for control of hyperglycemia during the acute stress period of a major surgical procedure.

More authorities have begun to advocate intravenous infusion of insulin instead of subcutaneous administration. Intravenous administration circumvents problems of insulin delivery in the event of peripheral shutdown (hypotension, shock), which might occur during major surgery. Furthermore, intravenous administration makes it possible to carefully control the amount and speed of insulin delivery appropriately based on frequent measurement of blood glucose. With either administration technique, the operative team should understand the management objectives and work together to achieve them. In this critical effort, it is particularly important to involve an anesthesiologist who is trained in the management of diabetic patients.

To assume responsibility for the management of patients with type II diabetes during and after surgical procedures, the clinician must learn specific techniques involved in preparing the patient for surgery and for managing the patient during and after the operation. These techniques are described in textbooks on diabetes (see BIBLIOGRAPHY).

The major principles governing the management of surgical candidates on the day of operation are presented in Table 3.12.

BIBLIOGRAPHY

Alberti KGMM: Diabetes and surgery. In *Diabetes Mellitus: Theory and Practice.* 4th ed. Rifkin H, Porte D, Eds. New York, Elsevier, 1990, p. 626–33

Arauz-Pacheco C, Raskin P: *Therapy for Diabetes Mellitus and Related Disorders.* 2nd ed. Lebovitz HE, Ed. Alexandria, VA, Am. Diabetes Assoc., 1994, p. 156–63

Medical Management of Pregnancy Complicated by Diabetes. Jovanovic-Peterson L, Ed. Alexandria, VA, Am. Diabetes Assoc., 1993

Proceedings of the Third International Workshop-Conference on Gestational Diabetes Mellitus. *Diabetes* 40 (Suppl. 2):1–201, 1991

Table 3.12. Major Principles Governing Management of Diabetic Patients During Surgery in Hospitals and Ambulatory Care Centers

■ General management goals are to prevent hypoglycemia and ketoacidosis, control hyperglycemia, maintain normal electrolyte and fluid balance, and resume oral feedings as soon as possible.

■ Management is considered satisfactory when random plasma glucose levels during and after surgery are between 125 and 200 mg/dl (6.9 and 11.1 mM). Clearly, the clinician in charge must make judgments about target plasma glucose levels, taking into consideration the skill and availability of the operative/postoperative team.

■ Plasma glucose levels should be determined frequently in the perioperative period as a guide to therapy; urine glucose levels are unreliable. The usual recommendation is to obtain plasma glucose levels every 4–6 h until the patient resumes oral feeding, unless severe hyperglycemia necessitates more intense management.

■ Mild hyperglycemia is preferable to hypoglycemia, especially during surgery. The actual amount of insulin used is determined by considering the patient's plasma glucose levels before, during, and after surgery, and, in the case of an insulin-taking patient, the usual insulin requirement.

■ Human insulin should be used to cover patients who usually are not treated with insulin because it is less antigenic.

■ Surgery should be scheduled for early morning, if possible.

Assessment of Treatment Efficacy

INTRODUCTION

In clinical practice, the therapeutic response to treatment of diabetes mellitus is, for the most part, monitored by determining effects on glucose metabolism. Specifically, the degree of blood glucose control is documented with various direct and indirect techniques employed by the clinician and the patient. In general, physicians assess blood glucose control with determinations of fasting, prandial, and postprandial plasma glucose levels and with assays for glycated hemoglobin. Patients can determine the effects of therapy with SMBG and measurement of urine ketones, if necessary. Some patients also keep a daily diary in which they record food intake, meal plan, doses of insulin or oral hypoglycemic drugs, symptoms, and the results of self-administered blood tests.

Monitoring of diabetes therapy should be commensurate with the various forms of therapy. The frequency of patient visits, for example, cannot be dictated. Most often, patients are seen fairly frequently after initiating treatment. In some cases, initial visits are used for the purpose of determining the degree of lability of blood glucose; in other cases, they are used to reinforce the necessity of following the therapeutic plan.

The selection of self-monitoring methods depends on the individual patient. Self-monitoring requires manual dexterity, cooperation, and intelligence on the part of the patient. Beyond that, the health-care team must consider the severity of the patient's illness and the patient's socioeconomic circumstances when recommending particular self-monitoring techniques.

Each of the assessment methods described below has advantages and disadvantages. Most often, a combination of methods is used to determine degree of metabolic control.

OFFICE METHODS

When a patient visits the office or clinic, the clinician can assess the degree of blood glucose control with a plasma glucose determination and an assay for glycated hemoglobin. Both measurements are of value: the plasma glucose is an index of day-to-day control, whereas the glycated hemoglobin concentration reflects the level of glucose control for the preceding 2–3 mo. The office visit is an opportune time to check the SMBG technique of the patient and address questions of meter use and calibration. In addition, it is important for the clinician to assess cardiovascular risk factors, including smoking and blood pressure status, as well as serum lipids.

Plasma Glucose Determinations

Fasting plasma glucose is an easily measured and useful parameter of metabolic control in a patient treated with diet or oral agents. It is not be as good a reflection of chronic metabolic control in patients treated with insulin. The major drawback to random plasma glucose determination, particularly in a patient with moderate to severe disease, is that it is difficult to know what a single blood glucose determination reflects. Even in patients with type II diabetes, blood glucose levels range widely during the day, so random determinations may simply represent peak values, trough values, or values in between. Furthermore, if the patient is visiting the office because of intercurrent illness, which frequently is the case, blood glucose levels will be of little value in that illness alters glucose tolerance. Also, some patients become more conscientious about following prescribed therapy just before office visits, in which case the random plasma glucose level may be misleading. For these reasons, plasma glucose levels should be supplemented at regular intervals (e.g., every 2–3 mo) with an assay for glycated hemoglobin.

Glycated Hemoglobin Concentration

Glycated hemoglobin is expressed as a percentage of total hemoglobin, i.e., the fraction of total hemoglobin that has glucose attached. Depending on the assay method used, the glycated fraction may be called total glycated hemoglobin, hemoglobin A_1, or hemoglobin A_{1c}. Although the different measurements all have different nondiabetic ranges, the results of all assay methods, when properly performed, correlate closely with each other. Clinicians should become familiar with the assay used in their clinical laboratory and its nondiabetic range.

A glycated hemoglobin concentration may be used to assess the effects of changes in therapy made 4–8 wk earlier. It should not be used in the insulin-treated individual to determine the need for short-term changes in treatment. Blood glucose levels are still the means by which hour-to-hour and day-to-day changes in insulin management are determined. Most diabetes specialists consider the glycated hemoglobin level more important than an isolated plasma glucose level for assessing glycemic control, because the latter is a single point in a fluctuating line and the former provides an index of the average. Furthermore, health-care providers have learned not to rely solely on SMBG results because the measurements are subject to errors in technique and the records are subject to errors of omission and commission. If indeed the glycation of other proteins is the basis of the microangiopathy and the neuropathy of diabetes, the glycated hemoglobin concentration may even be an index of the predisposition to these complications.

Certain conditions and interfering substances affect glycated hemoglobin results, depending on the assay method used. Any condition that increases erythrocyte turnover, e.g., bleeding, pregnancy, or splenectomy, will spuriously lower glycated hemoglobin concentration in all assays. In addition, hemoglobinopathies, e.g., sickle cell trait or disease, or hemoglobin C or D will falsely lower glycated hemoglobin results when hemoglobins are separated by nonspecific methods based on charge, solubility, and size (HbA_1 or HbA_{1c}). Other conditions, e.g., uremia, high concentrations of fetal hemoglobin (HbF), high aspirin doses (usually >10 g/day), or high concentrations of ethanol, may falsely increase glycated hemoglobin levels with the nonspecific methods. These artifacts do not occur with the more specific methods that measure glycated hemoglobin levels by affinity chromatography.

Measurement of other glycated proteins, e.g., albumin or serum proteins, has been proposed as another means of determining average glucose control. These methods, including measurement of serum fructosamine and affinity measurement of glycated albumin, reflect a shorter period (~2–3 wk) of average glucose control than glycated hemoglobin, predicated on the shorter half-life of serum proteins compared with hemoglobin. The shorter period of average glycemia reflected by the measurement of glycated serum proteins limits the utility of these methods, and most diabetes care specialists prefer to use glycated hemoglobin concentrations to monitor diabetes.

SELF-MONITORING

Between office visits, the patient can determine the degree of metabolic control by performing SMBG and keeping a daily record of test results.

Blood Glucose Monitoring

With the advent of SMBG, near-normal glucose levels have become a realistic goal for many patients with diabetes mellitus. Blood glucose monitoring is considerably more accurate than urine glucose tests for the detection of hyperglycemia and provides the ability to detect hypoglycemia before it becomes symptomatic. SMBG actively involves patients in the treatment process by allowing the patient to make adjustments in diet, exercise, and medication. Periodic self-monitoring is a valuable tool for increasing patient commitment to the prescribed therapeutic plan.

SMBG is particularly recommended for all patients on insulin and patients on oral hypoglycemic agents who are at risk for hypoglycemia. SMBG is useful for patients with mild diabetes during periods of stress, such as those caused by infection or trauma.

Frequency of SMBG will vary depending on the diabetes therapy. Most clinicians ask patients on insulin to monitor at least twice a day (before breakfast and before supper). Others ask patients to monitor more frequently (up to 4 times a day), e.g., before breakfast, lunch, supper, and bedtime snack. This is especially important for patients taking short-acting insulin alone or in combination with intermediate-acting insulin. In the subset of patients who achieve stable blood glucose levels, it may be appropriate to decrease the frequency of SMBG, e.g., before breakfast and dinner 2–3 times/wk. Well-regulated patients on oral hypoglycemic agents may show a pattern of decreased blood glucose levels in the afternoon that rise overnight. This pattern is best detected by SMBG and can be treated by appropriate medication adjustment. Many meters can be adapted for use by patients with visual impairment. The use of an automated lance for finger-stick is recommended.

Urine Glucose Determinations

The determination of urine glucose has, for the most part, been superseded by SMBG. Urine glucose measurements are indirect and imprecise, and they should be reserved for patients who cannot or will not test blood glucose levels.

Urine Ketone Determinations

Patients with type II diabetes rarely have ketosis. However, some experts recommend ketone testing in the presence of serious illness. Nonfasting urine ketones in a type II diabetic patient is a worrisome finding that requires further evaluation.

Patient Record

The patient should be encouraged to keep a daily record of food intake, doses of insulin or oral hypoglycemic drug, symptoms (including the time and circumstances), and results of all blood testing. This record serves to reinforce positive behaviors and to demonstrate their beneficial outcomes. Indeed, this type of record is important for the overweight individual, because the requirement to document food eaten during the day often helps patients to modify their eating habits and to initiate weight reduction. The daily diary is particularly important if the patient has labile diabetes or is taking insulin. It allows these patients to see the impact of diet, exercise, and drug/insulin therapy on glycemic control.

The patient record is helpful to the health-care team because it indicates the patient's degree of interest in control and provides information necessary for development of effective therapeutic plans.

BIBLIOGRAPHY

American Diabetes Association consensus statement: Self-monitoring of blood glucose. *Diabetes Care* 16 (Suppl. 2):60–65, 1993

Burritt MR, Hanson E, Murene NE, Zimmerman BR: Portable blood glucose meters: teaching patients how to correctly monitor diabetes. *Postgraduate Med* 89:75–84, 1991

Larsen ML, Horder M, Mogensen EF: Long-term monitoring of glycated hemoglobin levels in insulin dependent diabetes mellitus. *N Engl J Med* 323:1021, 1990

Nathan DM: Glycated hemoglobin: what it is and how to use it. *Clin Diabetes* 1:1–7, 1983

Self-monitoring methods for blood glucose. *Med Lett Drugs Ther* 25: 42–44, 1983

Promoting Behavior Change

Highlights
Promoting Behavior Change

Because the diagnosis of type II diabetes usually occurs in adulthood, lifestyle patterns and behaviors are firmly established. Optimal self-management of diabetes requires active participation by the patient in
- changing existing behaviors and
- adopting new behaviors.

The entire health-care team must assist the patient in behavior change. This process continues throughout life.

A successful program of behavior change includes patient education, skill development, and motivation to help the patient develop desirable behaviors, including
- healthy eating,
- regular exercise,
- taking diabetes medications safely, regularly, and at specific times,
- performing self-monitoring of blood glucose and utilizing the information,
- performing routine foot care,
- properly managing illness,
- developing a support system and coping skills, and
- utilizing the health-care system.

Individualized education and problem solving are at the heart of successful behavior change. The behavior change process is similar to the education process and involves assessment, planning, implementation, documentation, and evaluation.

Promoting Behavior Change

INTRODUCTION

The diagnosis of type II diabetes generally occurs at a time in life when specific lifestyle patterns and behaviors are firmly established. Optimal self-management of diabetes will require changing existing behaviors as well as adopting new ones. A successful program for behavior change requires comprehensive patient education, skill development, and motivation. This is best accomplished through a team effort. Physicians, dietitians, nurses, and other health professionals, i.e., the health-care team, should utilize their expertise to design a therapeutic regimen that promotes active patient participation in achieving the best metabolic control possible.

The importance of the health-care team in managing diabetes was clearly illustrated in the Diabetes Control and Complications Trial (DCCT), where the level of desired glycemic control was accomplished only through the combined efforts of a treatment team. Not only did each member of the team actively participate in patient education and skill development, but they were able to provide the regular and frequent follow-up identified as a crucial component of intensive management of diabetes. It is during these ongoing follow-up encounters that the most active level of education and support in the behavior change process occurs.

The knowledge and skills necessary to implement a treatment regimen cannot be acquired during a single brief encounter on the day of diagnosis. Change occurs gradually over time and generally occurs in small increments. It is not uncommon for patients to experience periodic setbacks where motivation wanes and barriers to implementing a behavior interfere with self-management of diabetes. This is when the patient benefits from the experience and availability of the multidisciplinary health-care team, which can provide not only specific problem-solving skills but also necessary support. A health-care system or environment must support these kinds of efforts if optimal diabetes control and subsequent improvements in patient health outcomes are to occur.

DESIRABLE BEHAVIORS IN TYPE II DIABETES

The goals of behavior change in type II diabetes encompass adopting a healthy lifestyle and performing necessary diabetes management tasks. Desirable behaviors will differ with each individual but generally involve:

- **Healthy eating.** For most people with type II diabetes, who are obese, modest calorie restriction and modifying eating behaviors to achieve or maintain even a minimal weight loss (10% of original weight) is a priority behavioral goal. All individuals with type II diabetes, regardless of weight, would benefit from following the Food Guide Pyramid for healthy eating to improve food choices. The focus in these guidelines is on including a variety of foods and not on deprivation. (See NUTRITION, pages 28–34). The American Diabetes Association embraces these principles of healthy, realistic eating behaviors. Nutrition therapy should help patients modify fat intake to reduce cardiovascular risk and modify food intake patterns to help reach blood glucose goals.

- **Regular exercise.** The benefits of exercise for people with type II diabetes are great, making regular exercise a desirable behavior. Blood glucose control, blood lipids, and general fitness are improved with a regular exercise routine that minimally occurs 3 time/wk. Obese individuals require exercise 5 times/wk to be successful at weight loss. (See EXERCISE, pages 36–39). Ideally, exercise should be both aerobic and strengthening. This can be a tall order for someone who may have spent a lifetime avoiding physical activity.

- **Taking diabetes medications safely, regularly, and at specific**

times. This may not be problematic for most individuals with type II diabetes but is sometimes a problem for the elderly. Individuals can fail to remember whether they took their medication, take the wrong dose, or deliberately not take it because they think they don't need it. Some elderly people with type II diabetes may become confused because they take multiple medications for coexisting problems. Healthy lifestyle goals include preventing and treating hypoglycemia.

■ **Performing self-monitoring of blood glucose (SMBG) and utilizing the information.** The discomfort and cost of performing SMBG is often a deterrent to patients with type II diabetes. This can limit the usefulness of SMBG in finetuning the diet or medication regimen. Clinicians need to make use of the SMBG data and teach patients how to use it to alter nutrition, exercise, and medication. (See SELF-MONITORING, pages 53–54).

■ **Performing routing foot care.** Older individuals are more susceptible to foot problems associated with diabetes and need to examine their feet routinely. Desired behaviors for proper foot care include smoking cessation, wearing well-fitted shoes, keeping feet clean, avoiding foot injury, and knowing what foot problems need medical attention.

■ **Properly managing illness.** Knowing how to maintain proper nutrition and hydration are important in managing illness in diabetes, particularly in older individuals. Knowing when to call a health-care team member is important in maintaining independence as well as preventing serious complications.

■ **Developing a support system and coping skills.** Stress can increase blood glucose levels. The diagnosis of diabetes and its daily behavior requirements, coupled with the usual day-to-day hassles of life, can be overwhelming. People with type II diabetes often have children, elderly family members, and demanding work schedules that leave little time for caring for personal emotional well-being. Having a support system makes the challenges of diabetes self-management easier to meet. Learning problem-solving skills, joining support groups, and educating family members about diabetes management are desirable behaviors.

■ **Utilizing the health-care system.** This includes keeping regular office appointments, following through with referrals to specialists and regular dental and eye examinations, and obtaining additional education as needed.

FACTORS INFLUENCING BEHAVIORS

Several factors have been identified as impacting the ability to change established behaviors. Age, socioeconomic status, and education level do not predict a patient's likeliness of adhering to a particular treatment regimen. Instead, focus needs to be on factors such as complexity of the regimen and the relationship that is established between the patient and the health-care team.

An individual's perception or belief regarding his/her susceptibility to the consequences of diabetes can also influence whether they can successfully adopt new behavior. This health belief model suggests that a patient's perception of the benefits and barriers that result from taking action influence their ability to change. Someone may, for example, feel that reducing fat intake to reduce cardiovascular risk is not necessary because they have had no problems and they don't wish to give up high-fat foods. The self-efficacy model suggests that, to make a behavior change, patients need to believe they have the ability to make the change with a reasonable amount of effort. For example, performing SMBG daily before breakfast and dinner may be possible, but doing it before lunch is out of the question due to work.

Specific patient coping skills may influence an individual's ability to change or learn new behaviors. Individuals diagnosed with diabetes may experience a range of emotions, from denial to anger, guilt, depression, and acceptance. Depression is generally more common in people with a chronic disease, including diabetes. Such emotions can immobilize a person in his/her efforts to actively participate in self-management of diabetes. Often, fear brought about by lack of knowledge is an underlying cause of the inability to act.

Characteristics of the behavior or regimen will also influence an individual's ability to change. The more complex a regimen is, the more difficult it is to adopt (mixing insulins vs. pre-mixed insulin preparations). The greater impact it has on lifestyle, the more likely it is to be ignored (exercising daily with a long work/travel schedule). If negative consequences exist (sore fingertips with SMBG), the behavior will probably not be as readily adopted.

Characteristics inherent in the relationship between the health-care team and the patient have also been shown to affect behavior change. Patients and their health-care team who share a mutual respect for each other are more likely to be successful at achieving self-management goals. This involves mutually agreeing on treatment goals and openly communicating regarding the barriers to achieving behavior change goals.

TECHNIQUES FOR CHANGING BEHAVIORS

Despite the many behavior changes required in managing type II diabetes, most patients can become successful self-managers of diabetes. Clinicians need to be sensitive to factors that influence whether a patient is ready and willing to make changes and then devise a plan to facilitate the desired change. The process of changing behaviors can take many forms but generally occurs in a stepwise fashion (Table 4.1). Individualized education and problem solving are really the heart of successful behavior change.

The behavior change process is similar to the education process and involves assessment, planning, implementation, documentation, and evaluation.

Assessing Learning Needs

The first step in educating an individual to make behavior change is assessment of knowledge, skills, and attitude. Current behaviors and lifestyle should also be thoroughly assessed. Generally, medical, lifestyle, and psychosocial data make up the assessment (Table 4.2).

Identify Desired Behaviors and Goals

Based on assessment, currently performed desirable behaviors can be identified. Most patients are doing some things well and should receive positive reinforcement for such behaviors. Desirable behaviors that need to be adopted can then become the focus. Providing the rationale for the desired changes helps the patient understand the importance of the behavior. Discussing realistic barriers to the performance of certain behaviors is important in setting behavior change goals with the patient.

Planning and Setting Goals and Objectives

The patient needs to be actively involved in setting realistic goals and selecting behaviors they are willing to change. This allows the patient to prioritize what is most important to him/her at the present time. Setting goals first focuses efforts on a progressive accomplishment of behavior change. Selecting specific behaviors is the second part of this process. Behaviors should be specific and measurable, e.g., walking 5 min after breakfast on Monday, Wednesday, and Friday. Choosing goals and behaviors that are within reach builds on a patient's self-efficacy and promotes further success.

Implementing the Education

Educating the patient by teaching necessary skills or providing the knowledge to perform the desired behavior in a format conducive to learning is critical to behavior change. The amount of information a person with diabetes eventually needs to learn is great. The National Standards for Diabetes Patient Education Programs specified 15 content areas. Actual content will vary with each individual based on their needs. Education can be survival level or more advanced. Teaching problem-solving skills to overcome a barrier to behavior change is an example of more advanced education (e.g., how to find time to exercise as a single parent with small children).

Various education strategies can be employed (Table 4.3). With older adults, it is common that family members are taught in addition to the patient or instead of the patient. Involving family members in the education process will promote behavior change by enhancing the support network available.

Documentation

Due to the complex nature of instructions and the need to inform other members of the health-care team, concise documentation of diabetes education is crucial. Appropriate problem solving through follow-up can only be accomplished with adequate documentation by health-care team members. Documenting goals and instructions for the patient is also helpful. Writing things down assists patients in remembering instructions and priorities. This can be a valuable education tool.

Evaluation and Follow-up

Monitoring behaviors allows feedback regarding the success or failure of a particular approach to modifying that behavior (asking the patient to record how often he/she exercises). Linking behaviors to specific goals such as changes in metabolic control reinforces behaviors. For example, measuring blood glucose after exercise shows that exercise can reduce blood glucose levels. Involving the patient in the evaluation is essential. Evaluation is done after a specified amount of time has elapsed since the initial goal-setting session. Routine office visits or phone/fax contacts can serve as excellent follow-up evaluations. Patients can fax or phone in blood glucose results that can be discussed and questions or problems can be identified and dealt with as they occur.

A crucial element in promoting behavior change is the problem-solving process. This is a skill that is best taught in follow-up sessions during those "teachable moments" when the patient perceives the need to learn and can utilize the skills to solve a real problem.

CONCLUSION

People with type II diabetes must incorporate numerous self-management behaviors into their lifestyle to successfully manage diabetes. Because these patients are usually adults, modifying behaviors must be accomplished using an adult approach that involves active participation by the patient. Health-care team members such as physicians, dietitians, nurses, and others provide the education and support to assist the patient in the behavior change that continues throughout the patient's life.

Table 4.3 Teaching Strategies

Methods
- Individual instruction: education can be tailored to individual learning needs and focused on specific details of patient's self-management plan
- Group classes: efficient use of educator time, patients benefit from social support and peer learning
- Self-study: flexible, allows patient to pace learning, educator should monitor and evaluate progress

Techniques
- Short lecture: effective for presenting new information
- Discussion: allows patient to personalize information, ask questions, disclose feelings, and share
  experiences
- Skills training: provides "hands on" learning: educator demonstrates, patient practices then demonstrates and receives feedback from educator
- Problem solving: allows patients to integrate information on several topics, such as diet, insulin,
  and exercise, and to test their knowledge in hypothetical situations
- Role playing: can be used to reinforce learning (patient plays educator role), to practice social skills (explaining diabetes to friends), and to explore personal problems (family stress)
- Case studies: provide and objective approach to learning that can be used for planning, problem
  solving, and to help patients identify errors they are making in their diabetes self-management
- Self-assessment: blood glucose records, food diaries, and exercise logs can be used to help patients recognize problems in their diabetes self-management and often to identify solutions.

Materials
- Printed materials: can be used to reinforce teaching, for self-study, and as an information resource
  for future needs (e.g., sick-day guidelines)
- Audio and visual aids: slides, films, overheads, audio and visual tapes, food models and labels,
  sample diabetes products, and dolls and puppets are effective in enhancing learning
- Interactive learning programs: available in printed, audio, visual, and computer formats; allow individuals to learn at their own pace, with frequent evaluation to provide feedback on learning
- Games: crossword puzzles, board games, and group games introduce fun into the educational process while enhancing participant learning.

BIBLIOGRAPHY

A Core Curriculum for Diabetes Education. 2nd ed. Peragallo-Dittko V, Ed. Chicago, IL, Am. Assoc. Diabetes Educators, 1993

American Diabetes Association position statement: Standards of medical care for patients with diabetes mellitus. *Diabetes Care* 17:616–24, 1994

Haire-Joshu, Houston C: Promoting behavior change: teaching/learning strategies. In *Management of Diabetes Mellitus: Perspectives of Care Across the Life Span.* Haire-Joshu D, Ed. St. Louis, MO, Mosby, 1992, p. 565–92

Meeting the Standards: A Manual for Completing the American Diabetes Association Application for Recognition. 3rd ed. Alexandria, VA, Am. Diabetes Assoc., 1991

Noninsulin-Dependent Diabetes: A Curriculum for Patients and Health Professionals. Ann Arbor, MI, Michigan Diabetes Res. Training Ctr., 1993

Detection and Treatment of Complications

Highlights

Introduction

Major Chronic Complications
Accelerated Macrovascular Disease
Diabetic Retinopathy
Diabetic Renal Disease
Diabetic Foot Problems
Neuropathic Conditions

Major Acute Complications
Metabolic Problems
Infection

Patient Cases

Highlights
Detection and Treatment
of Complications

Patients with diabetes are susceptible to numerous complications, both chronic and acute, as well as many adverse drug reactions.

The major risk factors for the macrovascular and microvascular complications of diabetes are
- hypertension
- hyperlipidemia
- hyperglycemia
- lack of exercise, and
- smoking

Most of these risk factors are more prevalent in the type II diabetic population and act synergistically to promote vascular disease.

MAJOR CHRONIC COMPLICATIONS

Men with diabetes are 2 times as likely, and women with diabetes are 3–4 times as likely as their nondiabetic counterparts to die from coronary artery disease. The average annual incidence of cardiovascular sequelae is increased at least twofold in patients with diabetes.

It is important to lower plasma lipid and glucose levels and to control hypertension, the latter being particularly important in terms of its benefits for reducing risks of microvascular (nephropathy and retinopathy) and macrovascular disease.

Hypertension is associated with increased incidence and rate of progression of diabetic retinopathy and nephropathy and, therefore, must be treated aggressively. Potential complications with antihypertensive medications should be considered (Table 5.2).

Nutrition planning and exercise programs should be utilized to help the patient achieve ideal weight. Cigarette smoking should cease.

Diabetic retinopathy does not cause visual symptoms until a fairly advanced stage has been reached, usually either macular edema or proliferative retinopathy. The changes involved in diabetic retinopathy may be subtle and suggest that all patients with type II diabetes should have a complete evaluation at least once yearly, including visual history, visual acuity examination, and careful ophthalmo-scopic examination with dilated pupils, by an eye doctor skilled in the examination of the retina.

A discussion of the clinical presentation of background and proliferative diabetic retinopathy is presented on pages 71–72. The indications for referral to an eye doctor are summarized in Table 5.4. Management of diabetic retinopathy is more successful when intervention is undertaken before visual symptoms develop. The ophthalmologic treatment of diabetic retinopathy depends on the stage of disease (page 73).

To monitor the onset of renal disease, a urinalysis (including microscopic analysis) and a serum creatinine should be done in all newly diagnosed patients beyond the age of puberty. Urinalysis should be repeated yearly in all adult patients. Urine albumin should be determined by 24-h (or overnight) urine collection.

Microalbuminuria usually is the first indication of renal disease. Consultation with a specialist is suggested if persistent proteinuria, elevation in serum creatinine, or hypertension inadequately responsive to treatment is seen.

More than 50% of the nontraumatic amputations in the United States occur in individuals with diabetes, and it has been estimated that more than half of these could have been prevented with proper care.

Early foot lesions often go undetected because they usually are painless. The prevention of foot problems requires proper foot care by the patient as well as early detection and prompt treatment of lesions by the physician. More serious foot problems are best handled in consultation with specialists in diabetic foot care.

The patient, with proper instruction, should assume major responsibility for prevention of foot problems. Minor noninfected wounds can be treated with nonirritating antiseptic solution, daily dressing changes, and foot rest.

The peripheral neuropathies include the symmetrical sensorimotor neuropathies of the upper and lower extremities, various specific mononeuropathies, neuropathic ulcer, and diabetic amyotrophy. Suggested approaches to management of these problems are presented on pages 77–78.

The autonomic neuropathies include gastroparesis, diabetic diarrhea/constipation, neurogenic bladder, impaired cardiovascular reflexes, and impotence in men. Suggested approaches to the management of these problems are presented on page 78–79.

MAJOR ACUTE COMPLICATIONS

The two metabolic problems of most concern in patients with type II diabetes are hyperosmolar hyperglycemic nonketotic syndrome and hypoglycemia in patients treated with insulin or sulfonylureas. Diabetic ketoacidosis may occur occasionally in patients with type II diabetes under severe stress (including severe infection).

The four major clinical features of hyperosmolar hyperglycemic nonketotic syndrome are
■ severe hyperglycemia
■ absence of or slight ketosis
■ plasma or serum hyperosmolality, and
■ profound dehydration.

Hypoglycemia can be precipitated by
■ exogenous insulin
■ oral hypoglycemic agents
■ decreased food intake
■ intensive exercise, and
■ alcohol and other drugs.

Hypoglycemia should be suspected in a patient who presents with manifestations of altered mental and/or neurologic function as well as adrenergic responses. The diagnosis is confirmed by a plasma glucose level <60 mg/dl (<3.3 mM).

If the patient is conscious, hypoglycemia should be treated by oral ingestion of some form of sugar. In the unconscious patient, parenteral glucagon or intravenous glucose may be necessary. Hypoglycemia may be prolonged in patients treated with sulfonylureas.

Detection and Treatment of Complications

Many clinicians consider type II diabetes mellitus a "mild" form of diabetes compared with type I diabetes because it characteristically has less labile glucose profiles and can often be managed satisfactorily with nutrition and exercise therapy or oral agents rather than with insulin. However, patients with type II diabetes are afflicted with the same litany of diabetes-specific long-term microvascular and neurologic complications as patients with type I diabetes (Table 5.1). Moreover, because type II diabetes generally affects an older-aged population, it is accompanied by a high prevalence of premature cardiac and cerebral and peripheral vascular disease, the risk of which is magnified two- to sevenfold compared with the nondiabetic population. The occurrence of these complications, which can result in loss of vision, renal failure requiring dialysis or transplantation, amputations, heart attacks, strokes, and premature mortality, causes the greatest burden to patients with diabetes and belies the notion that type II diabetes is "mild." Because type II diabetes accounts for >90% of diabetes in the United States, affecting over 13 million people, it contributes a major burden to health care. For example, type II diabetes is currently the single most common cause of new cases of end-stage renal disease.

This chapter reviews the detection, prevention, and treatment of long-term diabetes microvascular (retinopathy, nephropathy, and neuropathy) and macrovascular (coronary, cerebrovascular, and peripheral) complications that accompany type II diabetes. In addition, the acute metabolic complications of diabetes, including hyperosmolar hyperglycemic nonketotic syndrome and hypoglycemia and their management are reviewed. Finally, patients with type II diabetes are often treated with numerous medications including hypo-glycemic, antihypertensive, and hypolipidemic drugs to treat their diabetes and common coexistent disorders. The adverse effects of these medications and their interactions are also reviewed. Patient cases that illustrate proper diagnosis, prevention, and treatment of diabetic complications are presented on pages 80–85.

Prevention and treatment of the long-term complications depend on reducing or eliminating identified risk factors for the development and/or progression of complications. Risk factors for the individual complications will be discussed, and the benefits of risk-factor reduction will be presented. The Diabetes Control and Complications Trial (DCCT) demonstrated the benefit of good metabolic control in the development and progression of retinopathy, nephropathy, and neuropathy in type I diabetes. Although it is reasonable to extrapolate the beneficial effects to type II diabetes, no interventional trials in type II diabetes, similar to the DCCT, have been conducted. Moreover, the risk-to-benefit ratio has not been examined for intensive therapy in type II diabetes. Until such data become available, the risks and costs of therapy designed to achieve near-euglycemia must be balanced carefully against the putative benefits. Treatment should always be individualized, taking into consideration patient's age and prognosis.

MAJOR CHRONIC COMPLICATIONS

Accelerated Macrovascular Disease

In the diabetic patient, atherosclerosis involving the coronary, cerebrovascular, and peripheral vessels occurs at an earlier age and with greater frequency than it does in nondiabetic individuals and is responsible for 80% of the mortality in diabetic adults. Thus, the clinician should be on the alert for signs and symptoms of accelerated atherosclerosis among diabetic patients.

Early detection of complications is crucial so that appropriate treatment can be introduced before major morbidity or mortality occur. Although most diabetic patients experience the same symptoms of coronary, cerebral, and peripheral vascular disease as nondiabetic patients, clinicians should be aware that neuropathy and other factors may alter symptoms in the diabetic patient. Diabetic patients may have no or atypical anginal symptoms, such as exertional dyspnea, rather than exertional chest pain. In addition, cerebral manifestations of hypoglycemia may mimic transient ischemic attacks, and symptoms of neuropathy may need to be distinguished from symptoms of intermittent claudication.

Cardiovascular Complications

Studies have shown consistently that patients with diabetes mellitus have an excess of cardiovascular complications compared with nondiabetic individuals. In the United States, for example, those with diabetes are two- to fourfold as likely as nondiabetic individuals to die from coronary artery disease, and the average annual incidence of cardiovascular sequelae is increased at least twofold in patients with diabetes. Most important, the relative risk for cardiovascular disease in women with type II diabetes is 3–4 times greater than nondiabetic women.

Diabetes as a Cardiovascular Risk Factor

Type II diabetes is an independent risk factor for macrovascular disease. In addition, common coexistent conditions including hypertension, dyslipidemia (decreased high-density lipoprotein [HDL] cholesterol and increased triglyceride and low-density lipoprotein [LDL] cholesterol concentrations), and obesity are also risk factors. The pattern of obesity is important, with central fat distribution (waist-to-hip ratio >0.9 in men and >0.75 in women) associated with dyslipidemia, hypertension, and increased prevalence of cardiovascular

---

Table 5.1. Chronic Complications Associated With Type II Diabetes Mellitus

Vascular diseases
Macrovascular
- Accelerated coronary atherosclerosis
- Accelerated cerebrovascular atherosclerosis
- Accelerated peripheral vascular disease
Microvascular
- Retinopathy
- Nephropathy

Neuropathic conditions
Sensorimotor neuropathy
- Symmetrical, bilateral
  Lower extremities (most common)
  Upper extremities
- Mononeuropathy
- Neuropathic ulcer
- Diabetic amyotrophy
- Neuropathic cachexia
Autonomic neuropathy
- Gastroparesis
- Diabetic diarrhea
- Neurogenic bladder
- Impotence in men
- Impaired cardiovascular reflexes

Mixed vascular and neuropathic diseases
- Leg ulcers
- Foot ulcers

---

disease, independent of obesity. Other risk factors demonstrated in nondiabetic populations, such as smoking and lack of exercise, apply as well to persons with type II diabetes. Finally, renal failure and even microalbuminuria may significantly contribute to the risk of macrovascular disease.

Importance of Modifying Vascular Risk Factors

Although most studies demonstrating the efficacy of reducing cardiovascular risk factors, such as hypertension and hyperlipidemia, in preventing or ameliorating cardiovascular disease have been performed in nondiabetic populations, it is widely assumed that such interventions will similarly benefit those with type II diabetes. Therefore, clinicians should emphasize reducing these risk factors whenever possible. Unfortunately, drugs used to modify some of the risk factors and complications in type II diabetes may worsen other coexistent conditions/risk factors. For example, antihypertensive treatment with thiazides or β-adrenergic blockers worsens atherogenic lipid profiles and glucose tolerance. Treatment of hyperlipidemia with nicotinic acid may also worsen glucose tolerance. Finally, more intensive efforts to lower hyperglycemia with sulfonylureas or insulin may increase obesity and hyperinsulinemia. Clinicians must take care to select treatment regimens that do not worsen the overall risk for cardiovascular disease.

Hygienic measures, including weight reduction and exercise for obese patients with type II diabetes, are the most cost-effective and safe means of treatment and should be included in all treatment regimens. Successful weight reduction with a balanced diet will improve atherogenic lipid profiles, glucose intolerance, hypertension, and of course, obesity. Low-dose (325 mg q.o.d.) aspirin has been demonstrated to be effective in reducing myocardial infarctions in nondiabetic subjects in the Physician's Health Study. Similar benefits may accrue in patients with diabetes with relatively few adverse effects. For example, the Early Treatment Diabetic Retinopathy Study (ETDRS) demonstrated the safety of aspirin therapy in people with diabetes.

Hypertension. There is general agreement that control of hypertension reduces the development and progression of nephropathy and atherosclerosis. In addition, an association between retinopathy and hypertension has been documented in some, but not all, studies. Treatment of hypertension in patients with diabetes should be vigorous; however, the presence of diabetes may make the patient more susceptible to some side effects of drug therapy (Table 5.2). For this reason, there is disagreement regarding optimal drug therapy. Initial therapy may include an angiotensin-converting–enzyme (ACE) inhibitor, a calcium-channel blocker, an α-adrenergic blocker, or thiazide diuretics in low doses. The

use of thiazide diuretics and β-blockers is controversial because these may increase cholesterol levels, exacerbate hyperglycemia, and increase the risk of hypoglycemia in patients treated with hypoglycemic drugs (β-blockers). On the other hand, these agents are effective, inexpensive, and in the case of β-blockers, of demonstrated efficacy in secondary prevention of myocardial infarctions. The adverse effects of thiazide diuretics may be minimized when used in low doses, e.g., 12.5–25.0 mg/day. The goal for blood pressure control is <130/85 mmHg.

For patients with an isolated systolic hypertension ≥180 mmHg, the goal is <160 mmHg. For those with systolic hypertension 160–179 mmHg, the goal is a reduction of 20 mmHg. If these goals are achieved and well tolerated, further lowering to 140 mmHg may be appropriate. These goals may require use of more than one antihypertensive drug. The presence of autonomic neuropathy with postural hypotension may limit attempts to control blood pressure ideally. Male diabetic patients may be more prone to impotence as a side effect of certain antihypertensive drugs.

Lipids. In type II diabetes, an increased prevalence of lipid abnormalities contributes to accelerated atherosclerosis. Characteristically, triglyceride-rich very-low-density lipoprotein levels are elevated, and HDL levels are decreased. LDL cholesterol levels may also be increased. Associated obesity aggravates the lipid abnormalities. This lipid profile is the result of a combination of altered synthesis, catabolism, and clearance. A fasting lipid profile is recommended at initial evaluation (see page 10).

The National Cholesterol Education Program (NCEP) developed recommendations for the screening and treatment of dyslipidemias based predominantly on clinical studies in nondiabetic populations. However, they have adjusted their recommendations based on extrapolation of data in nondiabetic patients to apply to certain "high-risk" populations, including patients with diabetes. In general, the NCEP recommen-

Table 5.2. Potential Complications of Antihypertensive Drug Classes in the Patient With Diabetes

DRUG	POTENTIAL COMPLICATIONS
Diuretics	
Potassium losing (thiazides, loop diuretics)	Hypokalemia, hyperglycemia, dyslipidemia, impotence
Potassium sparing	Hyperkalemia, impotence, gynecomastia
Vasodilators	Exacerbation of coronary heart disease, fluid retention
Sympathetic inhibitors	Orthostatic hypotension, impotence, depression
α-Adrenergic blockers	Orthostatic hypotension
β-Adrenergic blockers	
Nonselective	Cardiac failure, impaired insulin release with hyperglycemia, hypoglycemia unawareness, delayed recovery from hyperglycemia, impotence
Cardioselective*	Blunted symptoms of hypoglycemia, hypertension associated with hypoglycemia, hyperlipidemia, impotence
Angiotensin-converting–enzyme inhibitors	Proteinuria, hyperkalemia, leukopenia/agranulocytosis/cough

*Cardioselectivity may be lost with high doses.
Adapted from Christlieb AR: Treating hypertension in the patient with diabetes. *Med Clin North Am* 66:1373–88, 1982

dations provide a reasonable starting point for the treatment of dyslipidemia in patients with type II diabetes, with the following provisos. *1)* All patients with type II diabetes should be screened for dyslipidemia during their initial evaluation by measuring a fasting lipid profile, including triglyceride, total cholesterol, HDL cholesterol, and LDL cholesterol. *2)* The increased relative risk for cardiovascular disease in women with type II diabetes and the common coexisting risk factors (e.g., hypertension) place the entire population with type II diabetes in a high-risk category. Although there are few direct data available to suggest a salutary effect of lipid-lowering therapy in patients with type II diabetes, the consensus of diabetes experts is that this population should be treated vigorously to reduce recognized risk factors. *3)*

NCEP Step 1 and Step 2 Diets may need to be adjusted to incorporate the elements necessary for diabetes therapy. *4)* Side effects from selected hypolipidemic drugs (e.g., nicotinic acid) may have a greater impact in patients with diabetes, which should be taken into account when prescribing these medications (see MANAGEMENT, Table 3.8, page 43).

The most characteristic lipid abnormality in type II diabetes is an elevated triglyceride level. In many cases, elevated triglyceride levels can be satisfactorily lowered by decreasing glycemic levels with nutrition therapy, exercise, oral agents, or insulin. Nutrition recommendations for these patients include a moderate increase in monounsaturated fat intake, with <10% of calories from saturated and polyunsaturated fats and a more moderate intake of carbohydrate. These recommendations might translate into a meal plan where <30% of calories are from fat, and 50–60% of calories are from carbohydrate. In patients with triglyceride levels >1000 mg/dl, a reduction of all types of dietary fat to reduce levels of plasma dietary fat as chylomicrons is necessary.

Acceptable borderline, and high-risk lipid levels for adults are given in Table 5.3. Patients without evidence of macrovascular disease in the borderline or high-risk category should be treated aggressively with diet, exercise, and glucose control.

If these measures fail, the addition of triglyceride- and/or cholesterol-lowering drugs, depending on the lipid profile, is indicated. Data do not support a specific triglyceride level that will reduce atherogenic risk in type II diabetes. However, a triglyceride level >1000 mg/dl is considered a risk factor for pancreatitis and should be treated with medication. Treatment of lower triglyceride levels with medications is of unknown benefit. However, the consensus of diabetes experts is that when fasting triglyceride levels remain ≥400 mg/dl despite dietary intervention and hypoglycemic therapy, lipid-lowering drugs should be used. In the presence of dyslipidemia characterized predominantly by elevated triglycerides, gemfibrozil is recommended. Nicotinic acid, although efficacious, may increase blood glucose levels and should be used cautiously. If the patient primarily has elevated cholesterol, bile-acid sequestrants or inhibitors of cholesterol synthesis are recommended. The bile-acid sequestrants, nicotinic acid, and gemfibrozil have all been demonstrated to decrease cardiovascular morbidity in clinical trials that excluded or had very few patients with type II diabetes. Whether the results are applicable to the population with type II diabetes is unknown. Nevertheless, in the absence of significant contraindications to their use, most diabetes experts employ these drugs to treat hyperlipidemias in type II diabetes.

Cigarette smoking. Cigarette smoking is associated with accelerated macrovascular disease, and the presence of diabetes in a patient who smokes will further increase that individual's risk. Ongoing efforts should be made by the practitioner to assist the patient in discontinuing cigarette smoking, including enrollment in formal smoking cessation programs, behavioral modification, and use of nicotine patches.

Treatment of Macrovascular Disease
Clinical trials that examined the efficacy of secondary interventions (after clinical disease has occurred) have often excluded patients with diabetes. However, clinical experience and a limited number of trials in type II diabetes suggest similar efficacy of medical and surgical treatments of cardiac, cerebral, and peripheral vascular disease as in nondiabetic populations, with several caveats. Antianginal treatment regimens and treatment of other risk factors after a myocardial infarction probably provide a similar benefit as in nondiabetic popu-

Table 5.3. Lipid Levels for Adults

RISK FOR ADULT DIABETIC PATIENTS	CHOLESTEROL (mg/dl)	HDL CHOLESTEROL (mg/dl)	LDL CHOLESTEROL (mg/dl)	TRIGLYCERIDES (mg/dl)
Acceptable	<200	—	<130	<200
Borderline	200–239	—	130–159	200–399
High	≥240	≤35	≥160	≥400

HDL, high-density lipoprotein; LDL, low-density lipoprotein.
From American Diabetes Association consensus statement: see Bibliography.

lations. Clinical trials such as the Norwegian timolol study have included a sufficient number of patients with type II diabetes to demonstrate efficacy of β-adrenergic blockade in preventing a second myocardial infarction. In insulin- or sulfonylurea-treated patients, the heightened risks of hypoglycemia with β-adrenergic blockade must be taken into account. Vasodilators, ACE inhibitors, and calcium-channel blockers can generally be used safely in type II diabetes.

Despite the generally more diffuse coronary and peripheral artery disease in type II diabetic patients compared with nondiabetic patients, bypass surgery and angioplasty are effective treatments.

Diabetic Retinopathy

The importance of frequent evaluation and early detection and treatment of diabetic patients with vision problems is illustrated by the following statistics:

- ~5800 new cases of blindness related to diabetes are estimated to occur every year in the United States, making diabetes a leading cause of new blindness among adults;
- >80% of all patients with diabetes have some form of retinopathy 15 yr after diagnosis;
- loss of vision associated with proliferative retinopathy and macular edema can be reduced by 50% with laser photocoagulation if identified in a timely manner.

As in type I diabetes, the development and progression of retinopathy is duration-dependent and associated with higher glycemic levels. Although more intensive efforts to control glycemia in the near-normal range in type I diabetes have been shown to prevent or delay retinopathy, it is not known whether a similar benefit will occur in type II diabetes. Attempts to normalize glucose levels, especially with low-risk treatments such as nutrition therapy and exercise, are appropriate. Although the role of hypertension in causing or accelerating diabetic retinopathy is less certain, control of hypertension is crucial to reducing risk for macrovascular disease

and should be vigorously pursued. Relatively fewer patients with type II diabetes develop proliferative retinopathy than those with type I diabetes; however, macular edema may be more common. In addition to retinopathy, patients with type II diabetes develop cataracts more frequently or at an earlier age than people without diabetes.

Diabetic retinopathy does not cause visual symptoms until a fairly advanced stage has been reached—usually either macular edema or proliferative retinopathy. Management is more satisfactory when intervention is undertaken before visual symptoms develop. Therefore, periodic ophthalmoscopic examination by a skilled practitioner is of crucial importance.

Types of Diabetic Retinopathy

There are three types of diabetic retinopathy: *1)* nonproliferative, *2)* preproliferative, and *3)* proliferative.

Nonproliferative diabetic retinopathy (NPDR). The earliest stage of NPDR is characterized by microaneurysms and intraretinal "dot and blot" hemorrhages. NPDR occurs in most patients with long-term type II diabetes. In many cases, it does not progress and has no effect on visual acuity. However, if the abnormal vessels leak serous fluid in the area of the maculae (which is responsible for central vision), macular edema can occur with disruption of the usual transmission of light and a decrease in visual acuity. It is not possible to visualize macular edema with direct ophthalmoscopy. However, its presence can be suspected if there are hard exudates in close proximity to the maculae. Circinate hard exudates near the maculae are especially suspicious. Any of these findings should prompt referral to an ophthalmologist with expertise in diabetic retinopathy.

Preproliferative diabetic retinopathy (PPDR). Certain retinal lesions represent an advanced form of background retinopathy. When these lesions are found together, the risk of progression to the proliferative stage is increased. The PPDR lesions include cotton-wool spots (also referred to as soft exudates), which are ischemic infarcts in the inner retinal layers; "beading" of the retinal veins; and intraretinal microvascular abnormalities, which are dilated, tortuous retinal capillaries or, perhaps in some cases, newly formed vessels within the retina. When any of these PPDR signs are found, the patient should be referred to an ophthalmologist for further evaluation.

Proliferative diabetic retinopathy (PDR). The final and most vision-threatening stage of diabetic retinopathy is characterized by neovascularization on the surface of the retina, sometimes extending into the posterior vitreous. These vessels probably develop in response to ischemia. The prevalence of PDR among type II patients who have had diabetes for ≥20 yr may approach 30%. PDR poses a threat to vision because the new vessels are prone to bleed, especially if they are stretched by contraction of the vitreous. If bleeding into the preretinal space or vitreous occurs, the patient is likely to report "floaters" or "cobwebs" in the field of vision. The patient who has a major retinal hemorrhage will experience a sudden, painless loss of vision. The proliferation of fibrous tissue that often follows PDR can lead to retinal detachment as fibrous tissue contracts.

Prevention
The DCCT demonstrated that, in patients with type I diabetes, intensive treatment that lowers average glucose levels to near normal will prevent or ameliorate retinopathy. It is not unreasonable to assume that this finding also applies to the type II diabetic population. No other treatment to reduce the occurrence of retinopathy have been demonstrated. In addition, because photocoagulation decreases loss of vision by ~50% in patients with PDR or macular edema, identification of patients at risk in a timely manner is a major means of preventing loss of vision.

Evaluation and Referral
The changes involved in diabetic retinopathy may be subtle and escape detection by direct ophthalmoscopy. All patients with type II diabetes should have an annual examination with complete visual history, visual acuity examination, and careful ophthalmoscopic examination with a dilated pupil. If retinal photography is available, it may be preferable to ophthalmoscopy. The indications for referral to an eye doctor are listed in Table 5.4.

Note that visual acuity changes are frequently related to fluctuating glycemic levels and corresponding changes in hydration of the crystalline lens. Thus, the presenting symptom in a new patient may be a change in vision. Likewise, a patient whose glycemic levels are suddenly decreased in response to proper treatment may experience visual acuity changes and should be forewarned as well as reassured.

The multicenter Diabetic Retinopathy Study and ETDRS defined three indications for immediate referral: *1)* vitreous or preretinal hemorrhage, even in the presence of normal vision; *2)* neovascularization covering one-third or more of the optic disk; and *3)* macular edema. The risk of severe visual loss within 2 yr for patients with any high-

---

Table 5.4. Reasons to Refer Patients With Type II Diabetes Mellitus to an Eye Doctor

High-risk patients
- Neovascularization covering more than one-third of optic disk
- Vitreous or preretinal hemorrhage with any neovascularization, particularly on optic disk
- Macular edema

Symptomatic patients
- Blurry vision persisting for >1–2 days when not associated with a change in blood glucose
- Sudden loss of vision in one or both eyes
- Black spots, cobwebs, or flashing lights in field of vision

Asymptomatic patients
- Yearly examinations
- Hard exudates near macula
- Any preproliferative or proliferative characteristics
- Pregnancy

Modified from Rand LI: see Bibliography.

risk characteristic is 25–50%, unless photocoagulation treatment is performed.

Treatment

The ophthalmologic treatment of diabetic retinopathy depends on the stage of disease. There is no commonly accepted therapy for background retinopathy other than improved metabolic control. The ETDRS demonstrated that photocoagulation slowed progressive visual loss in patients with macular edema by 50%.

Photocoagulation is considered the treatment of choice for patients who have proliferative retinopathy with high-risk characteristics, and it reduces the risk of severe visual loss by about 60%. Photocoagulation is used to stop neovascularization before recurrent hemorrhages into the vitreous cause irreparable damage. Sometimes photocoagulation is used to treat eyes with PDR before high-risk characteristics have developed. However, the risks of photocoagulation are such that usually only one eye is treated; treatment of the other eye is deferred unless high-risk characteristics develop.

When retinal detachment and massive vitreous hemorrhage occur, closed vitrectomy can be used to remove bloody vitreous and bands of fibrous tissue. During the procedure, clear fluid is infused to replace vitreous, and traction on the retina is relieved. In ~50–65% of cases, some sight can be restored with this procedure.

Patient Education

As the most important member of the treatment team, the patient must be fully informed about the possible visual complications of diabetes and their treatment:

■ The newly diagnosed patient should be told that diabetic retinopathy, which can cause vision loss, is a possibility and that it is important to report visual symptoms promptly.

■ The patient should also be instructed regarding the possible relationship between hyperglycemia and diabetic retinopathy, with emphasis on the necessity to adhere to the prescribed treatment plan for diabetes.

■ The patient also should know that hypertension may worsen diabetic retinopathy and that its diagnosis and treatment are important.

■ The patient with diabetic retinopathy should be informed that isometric exercises that raise intraocular pressure can aggravate proliferative retinopathy. He or she should also be informed of treatment possibilities (including photocoagulation) and the need for referral to an ophthalmologist familiar with the management of diabetic eye problems.

■ The patient who is visually impaired or blind should be made aware of and referred to vocational rehabilitation programs and other social services.

Diabetic Renal Disease

The prevalence of diabetic renal disease is at least 5–10% 20 yr after diagnosis in patients whose diabetes was diagnosed after the age of 30 yr.

Clinical Presentation

The development of diabetic nephropathy is asymptomatic, and its detection relies on laboratory screening. The usual course of diabetic nephropathy in type II diabetes is not as stereotypical as in type I diabetes, but nephropathy tends to progress through a number of defined stages. The first sign of developing nephropathy is the occurrence of microalbuminuria (>40 mg albumin/24 h). Whether microalbuminuria carries the same risk for the eventual development of clinical nephropathy in type II diabetes as it seems to in type I diabetes is unclear. As nephropathy progresses, "clinical" (dipstick positive, > 300 mg albuminuria/24 h) proteinuria occurs, almost always concurrent with hypertension. Eventually, nephrotic range proteinuria develops, followed by decreasing glomerular filtration rate with rising serum creatinine until end-stage renal disease occurs.

Conditions That Influence Renal Function

In patients with diabetes, there are several conditions that either precipitate the development of nephropathy or exacerbate the condition when present.

Hypertension. Hypertension may precipitate the onset or further accelerate the process of renal insufficiency or both. Virtually all diabetic patients who develop nephropathy develop hypertension.

Neurogenic bladder. Neurogenic bladder may predispose the patient to acute urinary retention or to moderate and persistent obstructive nephropathy. In either case, renal failure may be accelerated.

Infection and urinary obstruction. When these occur together, the risk of pyelonephritis and papillary necrosis increases, and this may result in a decline of renal function. Repetitive urethral instrumentation increases the risk of urinary tract infections. Infarction of the renal medulla and papillae can occur from ischemic necrosis and infarction or obstruction and is typically accompanied by fever, flank pain, anuria, and accelerated loss of renal function.

Nephrotoxic drugs. Nonsteroidal anti-inflammatory drugs, chronic analgesic abuse, and dye-contrast radiographic studies have been associated with increased incidence and acceleration of renal failure in patients with diabetes. Nephrotoxic drugs should be avoided, and dye-contrast studies should be performed only after careful consideration of alternative procedures.

Prevention

To monitor the onset of signs of renal damage, a urinalysis (including microscopic analysis) and serum creatinine should be done in all new patients. A urinalysis also should be done yearly in all patients. A timed 24-h or overnight urine specimen should be tested for microalbuminuria or the albumin/creatinine ratio determined. The finding of albuminuria or proteinuria should be followed by measurement of serum creatinine or urea nitrogen concentrations and assessment of glomerular filtration. If present, infection should be treated before the significance of the proteinuria can be determined. The presence of microalbuminuria may be the first indication of advancing nephropathy and, if present, should prompt aggressive treatment of even modestly elevated blood pressure. To delay the onset and acceleration of renal disease in patients with diabetes, hypertension must be detected and treated aggressively. There are potential complications associated with the use of antihypertensive medications (Table 5.2), and these should be kept in mind when instituting therapy. As with retinopathy, the DCCT demonstrated a decrease in development of microalbuminuria and clinical grade proteinuria with improved metabolic control. Whether this pertains in type II diabetes is unknown. Consultation with a specialist is suggested if persistent proteinuria, an elevation in serum creatinine or hypertension unresponsive to treatment is seen. Lower intake of dietary protein (to not less than 0.8 g/kg body wt/day or ~10% of daily calories) may have a role in reducing the rate of progression of nephropathy.

Patient Education

With regard to diabetic renal disease, the following patient education principles are suggested.

■ Patients should be told that the detection and treatment of hypertension is important because high blood pressure precipitates the onset of renal disease and accelerates its progression.

■ Patients should be encouraged to have their blood pressure checked regularly and to adhere to therapy when prescribed. Patients should also be encouraged to limit their intake of dietary sodium and to achieve and maintain desirable body weight for the purpose of preventing or modifying the severity of hypertension.

■ The symptoms of urinary tract infection should be explained, and the patient should be instructed to report such symptoms.

■ Patients should know why the treatment of hypertension and recurrent urinary tract infection is important.

- The patient with signs of developing nephropathy should be told about the course of the disease and the options for treatment with dialysis and renal transplantation.

Diabetic Foot Problems

More than 50% of the nontraumatic amputations in the United States occur in individuals with diabetes, and it has been estimated that more than half of these amputations could have been prevented with proper care. Therefore, the clinician and patient who are conscientious about prevention, early detection, and prompt treatment of diabetic foot problems can make a significant impact on this problem.

Causes
Foot lesions in individuals with diabetes mellitus are the result of peripheral neuropathy, peripheral vascular disease, superimposed infection, or most often, a combination of these complications. Usually, foot lesions begin in feet that are insensitive, deformed, and/or ischemic. Such feet are susceptible to trauma, which may lead to ulceration, infection, and gangrene.

In most diabetic patients with foot lesions, the primary pathophysiologic event is the development of an insensitive foot secondary to peripheral neuropathy. Loss of foot sensation is often, but not always, accompanied by decreased vibratory sense and loss of ankle jerk reflexes. Sometimes diabetic neuropathy is accompanied and worsened by other types of neuropathy, most commonly alcoholic or uremic peripheral neuropathy.

In addition to insensitivity, neuropathy may ultimately lead to a deformed foot secondary to tendon shortening (contractures), which leads to decreased mobility of the toes, abnormality in weight bearing, and development of classic "hammertoe" deformities. The combination of foot insensitivity and foot deformities that shift weight distribution promotes the development of foot ulcers. Neuropathy also causes decreased sweating and dry skin. If left

untreated, cracked and thickened skin can lead to infections and ulcerations. Neuropathic ulcers in the diabetic patient often go undetected because they are usually painless.

The sudden development of a painful distal foot lesion, usually secondary to trauma, may signify underlying peripheral vascular disease, which is associated with findings of decreased or absent pulses, dependent rubor, and pallor on elevation. The extent of the vascular disease and its potential for treatment by surgical intervention can be determined by Doppler noninvasive techniques and arteriography. Revascularization procedures, such as angioplasty and bypass, are often helpful in treating patients with severe disabling claudication (at rest) or nonhealing ulcers or to aid healing of a planned amputation. Unfortunately, surgical intervention is not always effective in individuals with diabetes because many may have diffuse vascular disease.

Infection is a frequent complication of both vascular and neuropathic ulcers. Studies indicate that these infections are often mixed and that gram-positive organisms predominate.

Prevention
The prevention of foot problems in a person with diabetes requires proper foot care by the patient as well as early detection and prompt treatment of lesions by the physician. Help from special health-care professionals (podiatrist, orthopedist, vascular surgeon, and experts in shoe fitting) is frequently needed.

Physician responsibility. The first step in prevention is to educate all patients and to identify those who need a special or frequent evaluation because of risk factors for foot problems. During the evaluation, the examiner should determine whether the patient has experienced foot problems or intermittent claudication since the last visit. The physician also should conduct a thorough examination of both feet, looking for the signs and symptoms of impending foot problems (Table 5.5), which include foot deformities and ulcers. The

Table 5.5. Warning Symptoms and Signs of Diabetic Foot Problems

	SYMPTOMS	SIGNS
Vascular	■ Cold feet ■ Intermittent claudication involving calf or foot ■ Pain at rest, especially nocturnal, relieved by dependency	■ Absent pedal, popliteal, or femoral pulses ■ Femoral bruits ■ Dependent rubor, plantar pallor on elevation ■ Prolonged capillary filling time (>3–4 seconds) ■ Decreased skin temperature
Neurologic	■ Sensory; burning, tingling, or crawling sensations; pain and hypersensitivity; cold feet ■ Motor: weakness (foot drop) ■ Autonomic: diminished sweating	■ Sensory; deficits (vibratory and proprioceptive, then pain and temperature perception), hyperesthesia ■ Motor: diminished to absent deep tendon reflexes (Achilles then patellar), weakness sweating ■ Autonomic: diminished to absent sweating
Musculoskeletal	■ Gradual change in foot shape ■ Sudden painless change in foot shape, with swelling, without history or trauma	■ Cavus feet with claw toes ■ Drop foot ■ "Rocker-bottom" foot (Charcot's joint) ■ Neuropathic arthropathy
Dermatologic	■ Exquisitely painful or painless wounds ■ Slow-healing or nonhealing wounds, or necrosis ■ Skin color changes (cyanosis, redness) ■ Chronic scaling, itching, or dry feet ■ Recurrent infections (e.g., paronychia, athlete's foot)	**Skin** ■ Abnormal dryness ■ Chronic tinea infections ■ Keratotic lesions with or without hemorrhage (plantar or digital) ■ Trophic ulcer **Hair** ■ Diminished or absent **Nails** ■ Trophic changes ■ Onychomycosis ■ Subungual ulceration or abscess ■ Ingrown nails with paronychia

From Scardina RJ: see Bibliography

clinician should also check the pulses (dorsalis pedis, posterior, tibial, and femoral), search for bruits, and determine vibratory sensation in the toes and feet.

Patient responsibility. The patient who has been given necessary information and proper instruction should assume major responsibility for prevention of foot problems. The patient (or family member, in the case of a patient who is impaired by morbid obesity or blindness) should be given instruction on how to cut toenails straight across and to inspect the feet daily for cuts, abrasions, and corns. The patient and family should know the importance of regular washing with warm water and mild soap followed by thorough drying. They should be instructed on the use of moistening agents such as lanolin and the need to avoid prolonged soaking, strong chemicals, such as epsom salts or iodine, and "home surgery." The potential hazards of heat, cold, new shoes, constricting or mended socks, and especially going barefoot should be emphasized to all patients—especially those with peripheral neuropathy.

Treatment
Minor noninfected wounds can be treated with nonirritating antiseptic solution, daily dressing changes, and foot rest. More serious problems such as foot deformities, infected lesions, and osteomyelitis are best handled in consultation with specialists in diabetic foot care. Infected foot ulcers often require intravenous antibiotics, bed rest with foot elevation, and surgical debridement.

Neuropathic Conditions

The diabetic neuropathies are among the most common and perplexing complications of diabetes mellitus. A complete dissertation on the peripheral and visceral (autonomic) neuropathies is beyond the scope of this guide. Instead, a few important points about diagnosis and treatment of commonly encountered neuropathic problems are discussed.

Sensorimotor Neuropathy
The peripheral neuropathies include the symmetric distal neuropathies of the upper and lower extremities, various specific mononeuropathies, truncal neuropathies and diabetic "amyotrophy."
Symmetric neuropathy. This common problem may occur in the upper extremities but is more common in lower ones. The distal, symmetric sensorimotor neuropathy is most often only mildly annoy-

ing to the patient, causing "pins and needles" paresthesias, noted usually at night and less so during the day and with activity. As the neuropathy progresses, hypesthesia develops, placing the patient at risk for trauma and foot ulcers. Some patients develop serious sensory deficits without having paresthetic symptoms. Absence of ankle reflexes and decreased vibratory sensation are objective signs of neuropathy. In a few patients, painful dysesthesias with burning or lancinating symptoms may develop. The painful forms generally wax and wane but may persist for years. They may be associated with anorexia, depression, and weight loss, so-called "neuropathic cachexia."

There is little evidence that any drug therapy is useful in diabetic neuropathy. The B vitamins have been used extensively but have not been proven effective. There are reports that treatment with tricyclic antidepressant medication such as amitriptyline, carbamazepine and phenytoin may be helpful in some patients with painful neuropathy. A topical cream, capsaicin, is variably effective. Aldose reductase inhibitors have not been approved for therapy in the United States. Aspirin or propoxyphene should be prescribed as necessary for pain. Narcotics should be avoided as the risk of addiction is high. However, these may be the only effective methods of pain control available.

Mononeuropathy. The mononeuropathies are asymmetric and abrupt in onset. Extraocular muscle motor paralysis, particularly that innervated by the third and sixth nerves, is the most noticeable of the cranial mononeuropathies. Patients can also develop peroneal (foot drop) and median or ulnar palsies. Spontaneous recovery in about 3 to 6 months is usual. Compression neuropathies, such as carpal tunnel syndrome, are more common in diabetic patients.

Diabetic amyotrophy. Diabetic amyotrophy is a neuropathy and not a primary myopathy. It is characterized by severe pain, wasting of the proximal muscles (pelvic girdle and thigh), and modest sensory involvement. It is usually asymmetrical and more common in men. Prominent features include quadriceps involvement, atrophy of thigh muscles, and absent patellar tendon reflexes. Complete recovery usually occurs in several months to a year.

Autonomic Neuropathy

The autonomic neuropathies, which usually occur in concert with peripheral neuropathy, include gastroparesis, diabetic diarrhea, neurogenic bladder, impaired cardiovascular reflexes, and impotence in men. Clinically, they tend to appear late in the course of diabetes.

Gastroparesis. The patient with gastroparesis may experience early satiety, nausea, vomiting, and abdominal discomfort secondary to delayed emptying or retention of gastric contents. Metoclopramide, in doses of 10 mg 3–4 times a day, or cisapride is often helpful.

Diabetic diarrhea. Frequent passage of loose stools, particularly after meals and at night, marks the acute phase of this condition. Diabetic diarrhea tends to be intermittent and may alternate with constipation. Diphenoxylate (Lomotil), loperamide (Imodium), and clonidine have been shown to be effective. Some patients respond to treatment with a broad-spectrum antibiotic such as tetracycline.

Neurogenic bladder. Neurogenic bladder is characterized by a pattern of frequent small voidings and incontinence and may progress to urinary retention. The demonstration of cystometric abnormalities and large residual urine volume are necessary for diagnosis. Surgical intervention may be required if the patient does not respond to conservative medical measures, because chronic urinary retention may lead to infection.

Impaired cardiovascular reflexes. Orthostatic hypotension and increased heart rates may occur when autonomic neuropathy affects the cardiovascular reflexes. Patients with orthostatic hypotension may find relief with use of 9-α-fluorohydrocortisone and compression stockings. If 9-α-fluorohydrocortisone is prescribed, the initial dose should be 0.1 milligram, and increases up to 1 mg should be made gradually. The drug should be used with particular caution in patients with cardiac disease, because it causes sodium and water retention and, thus, can precipitate congestive heart failure. Clonidine, a central α_2-receptor–blocking agent, has been used to treat this condition.

Impotence in men. Impotence is a frequent occurrence in men with diabetes and usually manifests as lack of a firm, sustained erection. In most cases, libido and ejaculatory function are not affected, although retrograde ejaculation may be another feature of autonomic neuropathy. Table 5.6 presents some of the distinguishing characteristics of diabetic and psychological impotence. The measurement of nocturnal penile tumescence (NPT) is sometimes used to determine whether the patient's erections during sleep are normal, borderline, or abnormally diminished for age. When psychological and endocrine causes of impotence have been ruled out, the implantation of a semirigid or inflatable penile prosthesis or the use of vacuum devices allows the patient to resume sexual intercourse. Intrapenile injections

Table 5.6. Differential Diagnosis of Impotence in Diabetic Men

TYPE	LIBIDO	ERECTION LOSS	NOCTURNAL AND MORNING ERECTIONS	SPECIAL PARTNER ERECTIONS
Diabetic	Normal	Gradual	Absent	Absent
Psychological	Decreased	Abrupt	Present	Present

Adapted from Kozak GP: Impotence in diabetic males. In *World Book of Diabetes in Practice 1982.* Krall LP, Alberti KGMM, Eds. Amsterdam, Excerpta Med., 1982, p. 108–12

Table 5.7. Factors Associated With Hyperosmolar Hyperglycemic Nonketotic Syndrome

THERAPEUTIC AGENTS	THERAPEUTIC PROCEDURES	CHRONIC DISEASE	ACUTE SITUATIONS
Glucocorticoids	Peritoneal dialysis	Renal disease	Infection
Diuretics	Hemodialysis	Heart disease	Diabetic gangrene
	Hyperosmolar	Hypertension	Urinary tract infection
Diphenylhydantoin	alimentation	Old stroke	Septicemia
	Surgical stress	Alcoholism	Extensive burns
β-Adrenergic– blocking agents		Psychiatric	Gastrointestinal
		Loss of thirst	hemorrhage
Diazoxide			
L-Asparaginase			Cerebrovascular accident
			Myocardial infarction
Immunosuppressive agents			Pancreatitis
Chlorpromazine			

Adapted from Garcia de los Rio M: Nonketotic hyperosmolar coma. In *World Book of Diabetes Practice 1982.* Krall LP, Alberti KGMM, Eds. Amsterdam, Excerpta Med., p. 96–99; and Podolsky S: Hyperosmolar nonketotic coma. In *Diabetes Mellitus.* Vol. V. Rifkin H, Raskin P, Eds. Bowie, MD, Brady, 1981, chapt. 22

of vasodilating substances (papaverine, phentolamine, and prostaglandin) have shown promise as an alternative treatment.

MAJOR ACUTE COMPLICATIONS

The major acute complications of diabetes include metabolic problems and infection.

Metabolic Problems

The two metabolic problems of most concern in patients with type II diabetes are hyperosmolar hyperglycemic nonketotic syndrome and hypoglycemia.

Hyperosmolar Hyperglycemic Nonketotic Syndrome

Of all diabetic comas, hyperosmolar hyperglycemic nonketotic syndrome is the most common in older patients with type II diabetes. When this condition occurs, it can be life threatening. Hyperosmolar hyperglycemic nonketotic syndrome sometimes occurs in people with

undiagnosed diabetes and in those with diagnosed diabetes after long periods of uncontrolled hyperglycemia.

Precipitating causes. There is almost always a precipitating factor (Table 5.7). Precipitating events include the use of drugs as well as other acute and chronic diseases (particularly infection) that increase glucose levels. Abnormal thirst sensation or limited access to water can also precipitate this syndrome.

Clinical presentation. There are four major clinical features of hyperosmolar hyperglycemic nonketotic syndrome:
- severe hyperglycemia (blood glucose >600 mg/dl [>33.3 mM] and generally between 1000 and 2000 mg/dl [55.5–111.1 mM]),
- absence of or slight ketosis,
- plasma or serum hyperosmolality (>340 mosM), and
- profound dehydration.

Typically, the patient develops excessive thirst, altered sensorium (coma or confusion), and physical signs of severe dehydration.

Treatment. The precipitating event should be determined and corrected as soon as possible while life-saving measures are employed immediately. Dehydration, hyperglycemia, electrolyte abnormalities, and the hyperosmolar condition should be corrected with use of appropriate fluids, insulin, and potassium.

Hypoglycemia
This metabolic problem occurs in patients with both type I and type II diabetes.
Precipitating causes. Hypoglycemia results when there is an imbalance between food intake and the appropriate dosage of drug therapy (i.e., oral hypoglycemic agents, insulin, or both). Exercise, intake of alcohol or other drugs, or decreased liver or kidney function can precipitate or exacerbate this imbalance.
Clinical presentation. Hypoglycemia should be suspected in a patient who presents with symptoms indicative of altered mental and/or neurologic function (changes in sensorium and behavior, coma, or seizure), as well as adrenergic responses (tachycardia, palpitations, increased sweating, and hunger). The diagnosis is confirmed if a plasma glucose level of <60 mg/dl (<3.3 mM) is found when the patient is symptomatic.
Treatment. The objective of treatment is to restore the plasma glucose level to normal. When the patient remains conscious and cooperative, ingestion of some form of sugar by mouth (e.g., fruit juice, sugar cubes, glucose tablets, or a solution equivalent to 15–20 g carbohydrate) is usually followed by rapid relief of symptoms. In the unconscious or uncooperative patient, parenteral glucagon or intravenous glucose (50 cc 50% dextrose or glucose followed by 10% dextrose drip) should be given. In the setting of hypoglycemia secondary to sulfonylureas, hypoglycemia may be prolonged, and patients should be observed and treated with intravenous dextrose for at least 12–24 h.

Infection

The rapid diagnosis and treatment of infection in a patient with diabetes mellitus is absolutely necessary because infection is a leading cause of metabolic abnormalities leading to diabetic coma. The more common infections seen in patients with diabetes mellitus and some critical comments about them are presented in Table 5.8.

PATIENT CASES

The following cases illustrate the most important points about diagnosis and management of the major complications of type II diabetes mellitus.

Case 1: The 51-Yr-Old Executive Secretary

A.W., a 51-yr-old executive secretary with type II diabetes mellitus of 15 yr duration treated with nutrition therapy alone (although she had a course of treatment with tolbutamide for 6 yr until 5 yr ago), presents with a 3- to 4-mo history of progressive exertional dyspnea and easy fatigability. She reports no chest pain, except for an occasional episode of nonspecific chest discomfort after protracted sexual intercourse. She has not experienced nocturnal dyspnea, orthopnea, or peripheral edema. She reports a history of smoking one pack of cigarettes per day for 35 yr. Her family has no history of diabetes or cardiac disease.

Physical examination reveals an obese woman with a blood pressure of 138/85 mmHg, a pulse of 88 beats per min, and mild background diabetic retinopathy. The cardiovascular examination shows a normal-sized heart without gallops or murmurs and good peripheral pulses without bruits.

Laboratory studies reveal a fasting plasma glucose level of 181 mg/dl (10.1 mM), serum cholesterol of 245 mg/dl, triglycerides of 200 mg/dl, glycated hemoglobin of 10.1%, and serum creatinine of 1.1 mg/dl. ECG and chest X ray are unremarkable.

Because of the progressive nature of symptoms, an exercise thallium study is performed and shows a cold area demonstrable only with exercise. ECG abnormalities correspond to the anterior wall thalluim defect.

Table 5.8. Infections That Are Common or Special to Patients With Diabetes Mellitus

TYPE OF INFECTION	COMMENT
Cutaneous Furunculosis Carbuncles	For reasons not clear, patients with diabetes mellitus may be prone to recurrent furunculosis and carbuncles. Unless vascular insufficiency is present, warm compresses may be used for treatment.
Vulvovaginitis (less frequently, scrotal infections)	*Candida* skin infection commonly occurs in warm, moist areas, particularly in the region of the genitalia (also on the inner thighs and under the breasts). This is particularly common in people with type II diabetes who are over weight or who have been taking antibiotics. These infections can cause extreme discomfort to the patient and result in breakdown of skin, which may allow entry of more virulent organisms. Good glycemic control and local supportive antifungal treatment usually will resolve the problem.
Cellulitis, alone or in combination with lower extremity vascular ulcers	To prevent the spread of infection to bone and the necessity of amputation, treatment of infected ulcers and surrounding cellulitis must be aggressive. Antibiotics effective against bacteria recovered from the site (both aerobes and anaerobes should be expected), as well as surgical debridement and drainage, should be used.
Urinary tract	Asymptomatic bacteriuria occurs in up to 20% of patients with diabetes mellitus; some suggest that it be treated. Certainly a patient with neurogenic bladder is susceptible to urinary tract infection and sepsis. Treatment is mandatory in patients with pyelonephritis. Patients with serious urinary tract infections should be hospitalized, the offending pathogens identified, and appropriate susceptibility tests performed.
Ear	Malignant external otitis is relatively rare, but when it occurs, it is most often seen in elderly diabetic patients with chronically draining ear and sudden onset of severe pain. *Pseudomonas aeruginosa* is the usual pathogenic organism. This condition is fatal in ~50% of cases. Immediate treatment should include appropriate antibiotic therapy and surgical debridement when indicated.

Adapted from Rabinowitz SG: see Bibliography; and Casey JI: Host defense and infections in diabetes mellitus. In *Diabetes Mellitus: Therapy and Practice.* 3rd ed. Ellenberg M, Rifkin H, Eds. New Hyde Park, NY, Med. Exam., 1983, chapt. 32

The patient is treated with a course of β-blockers and calcium-channel blockers with elimination of her symptoms. A weight-loss program and low-fat diet coupled with a supervised exercise program result in weight loss, improvement of lipids, and normalization of the glycated hemoglobin.

Three years later, cardiac symptoms recur and don't respond to adjustment of medications. Coronary arteriography is recommended and performed. During the procedure, the patient is well hydrat-ed, and a minimal amount of contrast dye is employed. Proximal lesions are identified in two coronary vessels, with no distal lesions and good runoff.

The patient was referred for coronary artery bypass surgery. Six months after triple-bypass coronary artery surgery, the patient was symptom-free and stable.

Discussion Points
■ Coronary artery disease is the leading cause of death in patients

with type II diabetes, who have a two- to fivefold increased risk of coronary disease compared with the general population. The presentation is often atypical chest pain. Myocardial infarctions in diabetic patients can be "silent" and occur without pain.

- Patients with diabetes often have involvement of more than one coronary artery. Contrary to popular myth, the lesions are often proximal and amenable to coronary bypass surgery. The 5-yr survival rates for diabetic and nondiabetic patients with equivalent degrees of coronary disease are nearly equal.
- Because of the risk of contrast-dye–induced acute renal failure, coronary arteriography should be performed under conditions of good hydration with a minimal amount of contrast material.
- Smoking markedly potentiates the risk of coronary artery disease, and patients should be admonished to cease smoking.
- The hallmarks of diabetic hyperlipidemia are hypertriglyceridemia and lowered HDL cholesterol, which usually are proportional to the degree of hyperglycemia and are only partially responsive to glucose control.
- In patients with type II diabetes, hypercholesterolemia is common, usually mild, generally due to an increase of low-density lipid cholesterol and usually responsive to good nutrition management and regular exercise, including weight control, control of hyperglycemia, and reduction of cholesterol and saturated fat intake.
- There is no evidence to suggest that patients with diabetes should be treated more or less aggressively with regard to surgical intervention. Medical treatment should be the first route, unless left main or left main equivalent coronary artery disease is suspected or present. Assessment of the efficacy of therapy may be problematic in many patients because of the lack of typical

angina. Repeated exercise tolerance testing may be necessary to assess efficacy.
- Although the impact of risk factor reduction on preventing or delaying the need for bypass surgery is unknown, the consensus is that vigorous efforts to lower cardiovascular risk factors are appropriate.

Case 2: The 48-Yr-Old Accountant

C.B., a 48-year-old African American accountant with type II diabetes of 10 yr duration treated with nutrition therapy and glipizide, presents for general medical care, having just moved into your community. His history is unremarkable except for some increased fatigability and nocturia. Physical examination reveals a blood pressure of 185/105 mmHg, pulse of 84 beats per min, and fundi with some arteriolar narrowing, a few microaneurysms, and hard exudates. The patient has mild cardiomegaly with a prominent S_4 but no murmurs. The remainder of the examination is within normal limits.

Laboratory studies show a fasting plasma glucose level of 205 mg/dl (11.4 mM), glycated hemoglobin of 9.9%, urinalysis with trace proteinuria, and a serum creatinine of 1.9 mg/dl. The ECG reveals left ventricular hypertrophy, and the chest X ray shows an enlargement of the cardiac silhouette. Repeat blood pressure measurements on three other occasions are 190/105, 180/100, and 183/105 mmHg. There is no postural drop.

Treatment was initiated with atenolol. In response to progressively increasing doses, the blood pressure fell to 155/95 mmHg and the pulse to 55 beats per min. Prazosin was added, and the blood pressure fell to 145/90 mmHg. With the addition of clonidine, blood pressure was satisfactorily maintained in the range of 125–130/80–85 mmHg. Insulin therapy was instituted with morning NPH. Adjustment of the dose to 45 U lowered the glycated hemoglobin to 8%. With this treatment, the patient felt well.

Discussion Points

- Coexisting hypertension is of major concern in patients with type II diabetes mellitus because it increases the risks of atherosclerosis, renal disease, and proliferative diabetic retinopathy. It should be vigorously controlled, particularly in the presence of renal insufficiency, because adequate blood pressure control slows the rate of progression of nephropathy.

- The objective of blood pressure control should be to maintain the blood pressure as near normal as possible (i.e., 120–130/80–85 mmHg) without postural hypotension.

- Diuretics are often used first in the treatment of hypertension. However, diuretic agents may impair endogenous insulin secretion and, thus, may exacerbate hyperglycemia in some patients. Diuretic use also may be associated with hemoconcentration, fluid and electrolyte imbalance, hyperuricemia, short-term dyslipidemia, and impotence. Diuretics in low doses may have minimal adverse effects while maintaining an effective antihypertensive action.

- Other antihypertensive agents that may be preferred for use in patients with diabetes include ACE inhibitors, calcium-channel antagonists, and α-adrenergic blockers. A cardioselective β-blocking drug (e.g., atenolol) or centrally acting drug (e.g., clonidine) may be used as second-line therapy. A cardioselective β-blocker does not impair glucose counterregulation unless used in large doses, at which it can also alter the patient's symptoms during hypoglycemia (i.e., decreasing trembling and tachycardia). β-Blockers may be less efficacious in African American patients. To promote patient compliance, the simplest possible dosage schedules should be used.

- Renal insufficiency in patients with type II diabetes (especially among African Americans) is a concern. Renal involvement generally begins 10–12 yr after diagnosis of diabetes. Annual urinalysis should be performed to detect renal involvement. If proteinuria is found, a serum creatinine or creatinine clearance should be obtained.

- In type II diabetes, the coexistence of hypertensive nephropathy is common. Treatment for diabetic and hypertensive nephropathy is similar. Lower intake of dietary protein (lower limit of 0.8 g/kg body wt/day or ~10% of daily calories) may have a role in slowing the rate of progression or renal disease.

Case 3: The 56-Yr-Old Lawyer

P.L., a 56-yr-old lawyer with type II diabetes of 8 yr duration treated with nutrition therapy and insulin, presents in your office for routine follow-up. When he undresses for his physical examination, he leaves his shoes and socks on. You ask him to remove them, and he replies that it is unnecessary to do so because his feet are fine. You insist. Examination of his left foot reveals a small (1.5 cm in diameter) painless ulcer on the plantar surface over the first metatarsal head.

Physical examination also reveals absent Achilles reflexes, decreased vibration over the great toes and malleoli, and generalized sensory loss over the feet, with a stocking distribution. Peripheral pulses are intact, and the feet are normal in temperature. Culture of the wound reveals mixed flora, and an X ray of the foot is unremarkable. The wound is cleaned, and the patient is placed on bed rest.

Discussion Points

- The feet should be examined frequently, especially in patients older than 40, those with diabetes of more than 10 yr duration, and those with a history of neuropathy, peripheral vascular disease, or foot problems. Such evaluation should include a history of foot problems, paresthesias, or intermittent claudication; inspection of the feet, toes, and toe webs for ulcers, calluses, cleanliness, deformities, and fit of shoes; palpation of peripheral pulses (dorsalis pedis, posterior tibial); and determination of sensation (especially vibration) and intactness of ankle reflexes.

- Patients should be taught proper foot care, including regular daily inspection of feet, cutting toenails straight across, not walking barefoot, washing feet regularly, using lanolin to prevent drying, breaking in new shoes slowly, avoiding heat or self-medication, and promptly seeking medical care for all foot lesions including calluses.
- A warm, insensitive foot (i.e., neuropathic and pain insensitive) is at greater risk than a cool ischemic foot that feels pain.
- Once an ulcer appears in an insensitive foot, there should be absolutely no weight on the lesion. Antibiotics and debridement should be used as necessary.
- Peripheral vasculature can be evaluated by a Doppler stethoscope, determining the systolic pressure index (ratio of ankle pressure to brachial pressure). Values <0.9 signify the presence of vascular insufficiency.
- Patients with recently healed ulcers or with insensitive feet should try to decrease activities that increase barotrauma (pressure) on feet. Well-fitted orthotics (specially designed shoes) can help redistribute weight and decrease friction over pressure points such as the metacarpal heads.
- Proper foot care is crucial in preventing recurrence of foot lesions.

Case 4: The 46-Yr-Old Registered Nurse

H.M., a 46-yr-old registered nurse with type II diabetes of 9 yr duration treated with nutrition therapy and insulin therapy, presents for routine follow-up examination. Physical examination includes a funduscopic examination through dilated pupils. This reveals multiple microaneurysms, "dot and blot" hemorrhages, some hard exudates, and a few soft exu-

dates. The patient is referred to an ophthalmologist.

Visual acuity is 20/20 bilaterally. The optic media are clear. Ophthalmoscopy confirms the presence of microaneurysms, dot and blot hemorrhages, and both hard and soft exudates. In addition, a few areas of venous dilation and some intraretinal microvascular abnormalities are noted. No maculopathy or neovascularization is seen. Photographs of the fundi confirm the above. A follow-up ophthalmologic appointment is arranged for 6 mo later.

Discussion Points

- Funduscopic examination is best carried out through dilated pupils by an examiner experienced in the diagnosis and classification of diabetic retinopathy. Patients should be examined annually. Alternately, fundus photoscopes (seven field) can be used for detection.
- Most patients with diabetic retinopathy, including proliferative retinopathy, experience no visual symptoms.
- Certain characteristics of diabetic retinopathy indicate a high risk for loss of vision, which can be lessened by treatment with photocoagulation. These high-risk characteristics are: *1)* new vessels and preretinal or vitreous hemorrhage; *2)* new vessel on or within 1 disk diameter of the optic disk ≥1/4 to 1/3 the disk area in extent, even in the absence of preretinal or vitreous hemorrhage; and *3)* macular edema.
- The risk of blindness can be substantially reduced with careful and regular evaluations for early detection and with appropriate use of current therapeutic tools.

Case 5: The 58-Yr-Old Contractor

N.C., a 58-yr-old contractor with type II diabetes of 19 yr duration treated with nutrition therapy and glyburide, presents for his annual physical examination. During review of systems, he reports progressive erectile failure of ~1 yr duration. He says the problem began with inability to achieve vaginal penetration, and most recently inability to achieve any erection. Libido persists, but the patient is quite discouraged about his erectile incompetence. He reports no morning erections, does not use any medications except glyburide, and rarely consumes alcohol.

Physical examination is unremarkable except for decreased vibratory sensation in the lower extremities at the great toes and absent Achilles reflexes. SMA-12 is unremarkable except for a plasma glucose level of 174 mg/dl (9.7 mM).

Urologic evaluation demonstrates normal genitalia but absent bulbocavernosus and bulbosphincteric reflexes. NPT studies show absence of tumescence activity consistent with organic impotence. Serum testosterone and prolactin are normal. The urologist requests psychological consultation, including psychological testing. Results are normal.

The patient was referred for surgical implantation of an inflatable penile prosthesis. Both he and his wife are satisfied with the results.

Discussion Points
■ Psychogenic factors are the major cause of impotence in both diabetic and nondiabetic men. Even when organic factors are present, many men have impotence due to a combination of psychogenic and organic factors.
■ Neuropathic impotence in diabetic men is usually associated with coexisting peripheral neuropathy. There is a higher incidence of neuropathic bladder changes in impotent diabetic men. The bulbocavernosus and bulbosphincteric reflexes are often absent in men with neuropathic impotence. Vascular insufficiency has also been demonstrated in diabetic men with impotence.
■ Neuropathic impotence is generally manifested by progressive erectile failure. Ejaculatory capacity usually is not affected.

■ The most effective test for differentiating organic and psychogenic impotence is the NPT test.
■ The implantation of a penile prosthetic device is a highly satisfactory and acceptable method for the treatment of erectile failure. Penile injections with vasodilators are also highly effective, although long-term use may be limited by patient reluctance or development of fibrosis at the injection sites. In these and other appropriate patients, the use of vacuum devices can be recommended.

BIBLIOGRAPHY

American Diabetes Association consensus statement: Detection and management of lipid disorders in diabetes. *Diabetes Care* 16:828–34, 1993

American Diabetes Association position statement: Standards of medical care for patients with diabetes mellitus. *Diabetes Care* 17:616–24, 1994

DCCT Research Group: The effect of intensive treatment of diabetes on the development and progression of long-term complications in insulin-dependent diabetes mellitus. *N Engl J Med* 329:977–86, 1993

Diabetic Retinopathy Study Research Group: Photocoagulation treatment of proliferative diabetes: clinical application of diabetic retinopathy, (DRS) study findings. *Ophthalmology* 88:583–600, 1981

Gundersen T, Kjekskus J: Timolol treatment after myocardial infarction in diabetic patients. *Diabetes Care* 6:285–90, 1983

Kahn CR, Weir CG (Eds.): *Joslin's Diabetes Mellitus*. 13th ed. Philadelphia, PA, Lea & Febiger, 1994

Keen H, Jarrett J (Eds.): *Complications of Diabetes*. London, Arnold, 1982

Klein R, Klein BEK, Moss SE, et al.: The Wisconsin epidemiologic study of diabetic retinopathy. III. Prevalence and risk of diabetic retinopathy when age of diagnosis is 30 or more years. *Arch Ophthalmol* 102:527–32, 1984

Klein R, Moss SE, Klein BEK: New management concepts for timely diagnosis of diabetic retinopathy treatable by photocoagulation. *Diabetes Care* 10:633–38, 1987

Levin ME, O'Neal W, Bowker JH (Eds.): *The Diabetic Foot.* 5th ed. St. Louis, MO, Mosby, 1993

National Diabetes Advisory Board: *The Prevention and Treatment of Five Complications of Diabetes: A Guide for Primary Care Practitioners.* Washington, DC, U.S. Department of Health and Human Services, 1983 (NIH publ. no. 83-8392)

Nathan DM: Long-term complications of diabetes mellitus. *N Engl J Med* 328:1676–85, 1993

Physician's Health Study Research Group: Final report on the aspirin component of the ongoing Physician's Health Study. *New Engl J Med* 321:129–35, 1989

Rabinowitz SG: Infection in the diabetic patient. In *Diabetes Mellitus.* Vol. V. Rifkin H, Raskin P, Eds. Bowie, MD, Brady, 1981, chapt. 24

Rand LI: Retinopathy: what to look for. *Clin Diabetes* 1:14–18, 1983

Rosenstock J, Raskin P: Early diabetic nephropathy: assessment and potential therapeutic interventions. *Diabetes Care* 9:525–45, 1986

Scardina RJ: Diabetic foot problems: assessment and prevention. *Clin Diabetes* 1:1–7, 1983

Seltzer HS: Adverse drug interactions of clinical importance to diabetes. In *Diabetes Mellitus.* Vol. V. Rifkin H, Raskin P, Eds., Bowie, MD, Brady, 1981, chapt. 40

Singer DE, Nathan DM, Fogel HA, Schachert AP: Screening for diabetic retinopathy. *Ann Intern Med* 116:660–71, 1992

Index

Index

About the American Diabetes Association

The mission of the American Diabetes Association is to prevent and cure diabetes and to improve the lives of all people affected by diabetes.

The American Diabetes Association (ADA) is the nation's leading voluntary health organization dedicated to diabetes research, information, and advocacy. Through the efforts of state affiliates, local chapters, and thousands of volunteers in more than 800 communities across the United States, ADA carries out this mission, educating and building public awareness about diabetes.

As a member of ADA's Professional Section, you access an important network of 11,000 professionals involved in all aspects of diabetes health care — from diabetes treatment and education to diabetes research.

ADA provides a wide range of services and benefits to its professional members, including discounted registration fees for scientific meetings and education programs at the local and national levels; a subscription to one of ADA's professional journals; discounts on the entire library of ADA journals and books; listing in the *Professional Section Membership Directory*; council membership; a free subscription to *Professional Section News*, ADA's quarterly member newsletter; and the latest *Clinical Practice Recommendations*, a publication of ADA's official policies on standards of diabetes treatment and patient education.

For more information about membership, contact:

American Diabetes Association
Customer Service Department
1660 Duke Street
Alexandria, VA 22314
(800) 232-3472 or (703) 549-1500

American Diabetes Association's Prestigious Research Journals

DIABETES
The world's most cited journal in the field devoted to basic diabetes research. Contains major scientific papers related to the molecular, biochemical, and cellular aspects of diabetes. 12 issues/yr.

Professional members: $50, US/Mex ($53.50, Canadian residents, includes GST)
$105 International

Nonmembers: $100, US/Mex ($107, Canadian residents, includes GST)
$155, International

DIABETES CARE
The best-read monthly diabetes clinical research journal. Presents research advances and articles on the latest clinical findings that relate to diagnosis, diet, exercise, monitoring, drug therapy, and complications and their management. Includes analysis and comment on what the latest findings mean for you and your patients. 12 issues/yr.

Professional members: $50, US/Mex ($53.50, Canadian residents, includes GST)
$105, International

Nonmembers: $75, US/Mex ($80.25, Canadian residents, includes GST)
$130, International

DIABETES REVIEWS
World-renowned diabetes investigators review specific topics in their fields and discuss the clinical significance of their own research. Each issue is devoted to a single topic and explores the hottest issues in the field in concise, review format. 4 issues/yr.

Professional members: $45, US/Mex ($48.15, Canadian residents, includes GST)
$65, International

Nonmembers: $65, US/Mex ($69.55, Canadian residents, includes GST)
$85, International

CLINICAL DIABETES
Newsletter geared toward professional with busy schedules. Presents in-depth reviews on important topics in diabetes treatment, plus medical and legal case studies and digests of current research. 6 issues/yr.

Professional members: $15, US/Mex ($16.05, Canadian residents, includes GST)
$21, International

Nonmembers: $20, US/Mex ($21.14, Canadian residents, includes GST)
$26, International

DIABETES SPECTRUM

Concise, ready-to-use resource for diabetes educators and counselors that supports you in counseling patients with diabetes. Translates the latest clinical findings into practical strategies, techniques, and materials you can use immediately to help your patients. 6 issues/yr.

Professional members: $15, US/Mex ($16.05, Canadian residents, includes GST)
$30, International

Nonmembers: $30, US/Mex ($32.10, Canadian residents, includes GST)
$45, International

For more information about subscriptions or if you would like to find out more about **Professional Section Membership**, please call our Customer Service Department at (800) 232-3472 or (703) 549-1500.

Additional Resources From the Clinical Education Series

NEW!

Medical Management of Insulin-Dependent (Type I) Diabetes
formerly: Physician's Guide to Insulin-Dependent (Type I) Diabetes

The result of 10+ years of research and the expertise of the world's leading authorities on type I diabetes. This completely revised and updated edition features:

■ Revised Diagnosis and Classification Criteria
■ Updated Information on Pathogenesis
■ New Strategies for Achieving Better Metabolic Control
■ New Information on Preventing and Treating Diabetes Complications

Since the announcement of the DCCT results, it's now more important than ever to keep up with the latest developments in diabetes management. This book will help you translate these advances into superior patient care. And its succinct, readable format and thorough index make it easy to find the information you need in seconds! 1994. Softcover. #PMMT1
Nonmember: $37.50; Member: $29.95

NEW!

Therapy for Diabetes Mellitus and Related Disorders, 2nd Edition

Put the knowledge of more than 50 diabetes experts right at your fingertips! Updated to reflect DCCT findings and new treatment recommendations, each chapter focuses on a different aspect of diabetes and its complications, presenting a concise, practical approach to treatment. Contains cutting edge treatment information, including: the latest drug therapies; treating diabetic nerve, eye, and kidney disorders; psychosocial issues; managing ketoacidosis and hyperglycemic hyperosmolar coma; cardiovascular complications; and much more! 1994. Softcover. #PMTDRD2
Nonmember: $34.50; Member: $27.50

Medical Management of Pregnancy Complicated by Diabetes

A must-read for anyone involved in treating women with type I, type II, or gestational diabetes! This concise, yet comprehensive guide takes you through every aspect of pregnancy and diabetes, from prepregnancy counseling to postpartum follow-up and everything in between. Provides precise protocols for treatment of both preexisting and gestational diabetes. Tabbed and well indexed for easy access to important information. 1993. Softcover; 136 pages. #PMMPCD
Nonmember: $37.50; Member: $29.95

Cardiovascular Risk Factor Management: A Lecture Program

This 3-hour program focuses on diabetes and its complications as risk factors for atherosclerotic vascular disease. Covers epidemiology, pathophysiology, assessment, and treatment for each risk factor. Includes case-study discussion and presenter's script. 1993. 92 color slides. #PMCEP3SS
Nonmember: $250.00; Member: $200.00

Managing Diabetes in the '90s: A Lecture Program

Developed to give students a basic overview of diabetes, this color slide program discusses the screening, diagnosis, and management of type I, type II, and gestational diabetes mellitus. The accompanying presenter's script includes case studies and a hard copy of each slide. 83 slides. #PMCEPSS
Nonmember: $95.00; Member: $75.00

Nutrition Guide for Professionals: Diabetes Education and Meal Planning

This publication helps you effectively use the *Exchange Lists for Meal Planning* to create individualized meal plans for your patients. This book is vital to helping you understand the critical role nutrition plays in diabetes management. It also expands on the meal-planning model to include alternatives to the exchange system. Softcover. #PNNG
Nonmember: $12.95; Member: $11.00

Diabetic Foot Care

Prepared by the ADA Council on Foot Care, this booklet contains important information about preventing and treating serious foot problems caused by diabetes. Left unchecked, these problems frequently lead to amputations—something you and your patients both want to avoid if possible. Emphasizes educating patients about proper foot care and routine evaluations to catch problems before they progress. Softcover. #PMFOOT
Nonmember: $5.75; Member: $4.50

Order These Valuable Publications Today!

Yes! Please send me:

		Qty.	Price	Total
Medical Management of Type I Diabetes	#PMMT1_____		@$_____	each = $_____
Medical Management of Type II Diabetes	#PMMT2_____		@$_____	each = $_____
Therapy for Diabetes Mellitus, 2nd Edition	#PMTDRD2_____		@$_____	each = $_____
Medical Management of Pregnancy Complicated by Diabetes	#PMMPCD_____		@$_____	each = $_____
Cardiovascular Risk Factor Management	#PMCEP3SS_____		@$_____	each = $_____
Managing Diabetes in the '90s	#PMCEPSS_____		@$_____	each = $_____
Nutrition Guide for Professionals	#PNNG_____		@$_____	each = $_____
Diabetic Foot Care	#PMFOOT_____		@$_____	each = $_____

Publications Subtotal: $_____

VA Residents Add 4.5% Sales Tax: $_____

Shipping & Handling (based on subtotal): $_____

Grand Total: $_____

Allow 2–3 weeks for shipment. Add $3.00 to shipping & handling for each additional shipping address. Add $15 to shipping & handling for each international shipment. Foreign orders must be paid in U.S. funds, drawn on a U.S. bank. Prices subject to change without notice.

Name_____

Address_____

City/State/Zip_____

Payment enclosed (check or money order) OR

Charge my: ❏ VISA ❏ MC ❏ AMEX

Account #_____

Signature_____ Exp. Date_____

Shipping & Handling Chart
up to $30.00 . . . . . .add $3.00
$30.01–$50.00   . . .add $4.00
over $50.00 . . . . . .add 8% of order

Mail to:

American Diabetes Association
1970 Chain Bridge Road PH79402
McLean, VA 22109-0592

Order These Valuable Publications Today!

Yes! Please send me:

		Qty.	Price	Total
Medical Management of Type I Diabetes	#PMMT1_____	@$_____each = $_____		
Medical Management of Type II Diabetes	#PMMT2_____	@$_____each = $_____		
Therapy for Diabetes Mellitus, 2nd Edition	#PMTDRD2_____	@$_____each = $_____		
Medical Management of Pregnancy Complicated by Diabetes	#PMMPCD_____	@$_____each = $_____		
Cardiovascular Risk Factor Management	#PMCEP3SS_____	@$_____each = $_____		
Managing Diabetes in the '90s	#PMCEPSS_____	@$_____each = $_____		
Nutrition Guide for Professionals	#PNNG_____	@$_____each = $_____		
Diabetic Foot Care	#PMFOOT_____	@$_____each = $_____		

Publications Subtotal: $_____

VA Residents Add 4.5% Sales Tax: $_____

Shipping & Handling (based on subtotal): $_____

Grand Total: $_____

Allow 2–3 weeks for shipment. Add $3.00 to shipping & handling for each additional shipping address. Add $15 to shipping & handling for each international shipment. Foreign orders must be paid in U.S. funds, drawn on a U.S. bank. Prices subject to change without notice.

Name_____

Address_____

City/State/Zip_____

Payment enclosed (check or money order) OR

Charge my: ❏ VISA ❏ MC ❏ AMEX

Account #_____

Signature_____ Exp. Date_____

Shipping & Handling Chart
up to $30.00 . . . . . .add $3.00
$30.01–$50.00 . . .add $4.00
over $50.00 . . . . . .add 8% of order

Mail to:

American Diabetes Association
1970 Chain Bridge Road PH79402
McLean, VA 22109-0592